KNEE PAIN
and Disability

EDITION 2

KNEE PAIN
and Disability

RENE CAILLIET, M.D.

Professor and Chairman
Department of Rehabilitative Medicine
University of Southern California
School of Medicine
Los Angeles, California

Illustrations by R. Caillet, M.D.

 F. A. DAVIS COMPANY • Philadelphia

Also by Rene Cailliet

Low Back Pain Syndrome
Shoulder Pain
Neck and Arm Pain
Soft Tissue Pain and Disability
Hand Pain and Impairment
Foot and Ankle Pain

Library of Congress Cataloging in Publication Data
Cailliet, Rene.
  Knee pain and disability.

  Includes bibliographies and index.
  1. Knee—Wounds and injuries. 2. Knee—Abnormalities.
3. Knee—Diseases. 4. Pain. I. Title. [DNLM:
1. Knee. 2. Knee injuries. WE 870 C134k]
RD561.C34   1983   617'.582   82-17296
ISBN 0-8036-1621-X

Preface

The human knee is subjected daily to numerous stresses, injuries, and diseases, and it places high in the percentage of patients disabled from musculoskeletal impairment in comparison with lumbrosacral pain, neck and shoulder pain, foot pain, and hand impairment. As stated in Chapter One, the knee is probably the most complicated joint in the human body.

Therefore, this book is offered in an effort to acquaint the student, intern, resident, family practitioner, and nonorthopedist with basic knee conditions they may see, often in the early phase of pain or disability. As in the previous CAILLIET PAIN SERIES, functional anatomy is stressed and illustrations are schematic for simplification and economy.

In order to maintain the small size of this book, neither exhaustive presentations of the subjects that are discussed in this book nor *all* knee conditions can be included. New forms of treatment constantly emerge and new concepts of disease and disability become clarified daily by continuing research and clinical experience. Only constant study can keep the practicing physician and therapist abreast of advancing scientific knowledge.

This new edition contains additional material relating to ligaments, cartilage, and gait mechanisms. New sections include ligamentous capsular injuries and patellofemoral arthralgia. Sections on nonsurgical treatment have been expanded upon. Thirty-one new illustrations have also been added.

It is hoped that this book will lead to earlier recognition of knee conditions, better evaluation, increased physiologic treatment, and earlier referral for more definitive and specialized treatment when so recognized.

RENE CAILLIET, M.D.

v

Contents

Illustrations

CHAPTER 1

Structural Anatomy

The knee joint is probably the most complicated joint in the human body. It is intricate because its function is related to its gross bony anatomy, integrated muscular activity, and precise restrictive ligamentous structures. Its articular surfaces frequently are exposed to stresses and strains. Because of the knee's complexity and frequency to pain, a thorough knowledge of functional anatomy is mandatory for a meaningful examination, proper evaluation of symptoms and findings, and a physiologic basis for treatment.

OSSEOUS COMPONENTS

The joint is formed by the distal end of the femur and the proximal end of the tibia with interposed menisci, which give symmetry to the joint and aid in lubrication. Ligaments and muscles surround the joint. Motion is basically that of flexion and extension with minimal rotatory motion. The human knee, unlike that of lower primates, is capable of full extension (0°) and greater than 90° flexion. Slight abduction and adduction are physiologically possible with the tibia fully extended upon the femur.

The joint surface of the distal femur has two surfaces (Fig. 1): anteriorly, the femoral patellar and inferiorly, the tibial. The patellar surface is saddle-shaped and asymmetrical, with the lateral face larger and more convex than the medial plate. Upon this surface glides the patella, an integral part of the knee extensor mechanism.

The tibial surface of the femur viewed laterally is flattened in its anterior surface and curved on its posterior lateral aspect. The inferior surface of the femur is formed by two condyles separated by a deep U-shaped notch, the intercondylar fossa. This fossa is deep and wide, equal in size to that of a thumb. The medial femoral condyle has a smaller transverse diameter (TM in Fig. 1) but a longer longitudinal diameter (LM in Fig. 1) because of its curved direction. These condylar surfaces correspond to similar articular surfaces of the opposing tibial condyles.

1

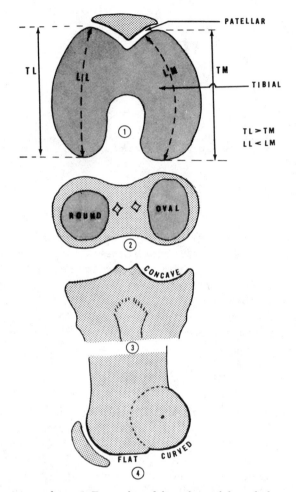

FIGURE 1. Knee joint surfaces. *1*, Femoral condyle surfaces of the right knee. *TL*, Anteroposterior length of the lateral condyle; *TM*, Length of the medial condyle. The length of the medial condyle *(LM)* is greater than the length of the lateral condyle *(LL)* because of its curved surface. *2*, Superior surface of the right tibia. The lateral articular surface is rounded and the medial articular surface is oval. *3*, The medial tibial articular surface is deeper and more concave than is the lateral. *4*, Side view of the femur showing the flat anterior surface and the curved posterior surface. The two articulations are illustrated in *1*: the patellar surface in which the patella articulates with the anterior femur and the tibial surface then glides upon the tibia.

The tibial plateau has two articular surfaces (see Fig. 1). Viewed in an anteroposterior direction, the medial surface is oval, deeper, and more concave than its lateral and rounder counterpart. The two surfaces arch upward toward each other and are separated by two bony spines, the eminentia intercondylaris (Fig. 2).

2

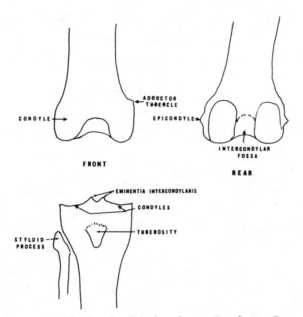

FRONT

REAR

FIGURE 2. Superficial landmarks of the knee bones. *Top*, femur; *Bottom*, tibia.

All articular surfaces of the femoral condyles, the tibial condyles, and the dorsal aspect of the patella are covered by cartilage with a thickness of 3 to 4 mm.

The joint capsule is large, permitting injection of 30 to 40 ml of air before causing tension. The capsule attaches to the femur near the margins of the articular cartilage at the site of the epicondyles. It is attached upon the tibia just distal to the attachment of the collateral ligaments. In the joint, the synovial membrane passes anteriorly to the cruciate ligament, thus making the cruciate ligaments *inter*articular but *extra*capsular (Fig. 3).

MENISCI

The asymmetry of the relationship of the femoral condyles to the tibial condyles is compensated by the interposed menisci. These are curved, wedge-shaped, fibrocartilaginous structures that lie between the opposing articular surfaces. They are connected to each other and to the joint capsule. These menisci assist in distributing the pressure between the femur and the tibia, increase the elasticity of the joint, and assist in its lubrication.

The medial meniscus is approximately 10 mm wide with its posterior horn wider than the middle portion (Fig. 4). The medial meniscus has a wider curve than the lateral meniscus. Its anterior horn connects to the

3

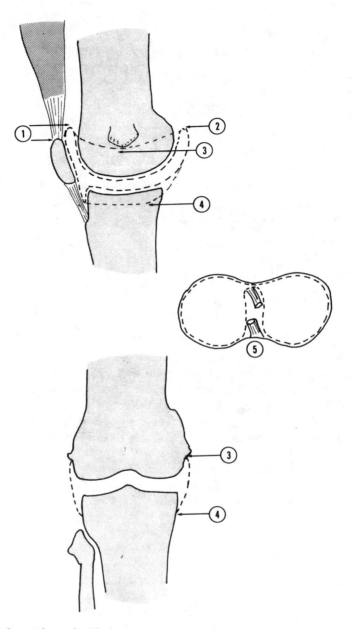

Figure 3. Synovial capsule. The knee joint capsule is large and shallow and can hold up to 40 ml of air without tension. *1*, Anteriorly, it ascends to two finger breadths above the patella. *2*, Posteriorly, it ascends to the origin of the gastrocnemius muscle. *3*, Laterally, it attaches to the femur at the junction of the condylar cartilage at the epicondylar level. *4*, Inferiorly, it attaches upon the tibia a quarter inch below the articular margin at the attachment of the collateral ligament. *5*, The cruciate ligaments invaginate the capsule; thus they are *extra*capsular.

4

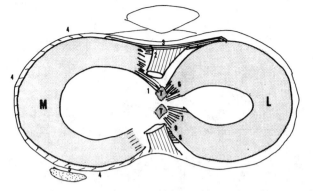

FIGURE 4. Attachments of the menisci. Right tibial plateau viewed from above. *1*, Fibrous attachment of the medial meniscus *(M)* to outer ridge of the tibial tubercle *(T)*. *2*, Connection to the anterior cruciate ligament and *(3)* to the anterior horn of the lateral meniscus *(L)* via the ligamentous transversus. *4*, The medial meniscus is attached around its entire periphery to the capsule and *(5)* posteriorly to the semimembranosus muscle tendon. The lateral meniscus has both its *(6)* anterior and *(7)* posterior horns attached to the eminentia intercondylaris *(T)* by a fibrous connection *(8)* to the posterior cruciate ligament. *(9)*, A fibrous band attaches superiorly into the fossa intercondylaris of the femur.

anterior ridge of the tibia by fibrous ligamentous tissue and to the ventral intercondylar spine. It often connects with the anterior cruciate ligament. By way of the ligamentous transversus, it connects to the anterior horn of the lateral meniscus. Around its outer periphery, it is firmly connected to the joint capsule and the medial collateral ligament. Posteriorly, the medial meniscus connects to a fibrous thickening of the capsule and is connected to the tendinous portion of the semimembranous muscle.

The lateral meniscus has a width of 12 to 13 mm. Its curvature is greater than the medial meniscus, causing it to resemble a closed ring. Both the anterior and posterior horns of the lateral meniscus insert directly into the eminentia intercondylaris and by a fibrous connnection to the posterior cruciate ligament, the ligamentous menisci fibularis. Most of the posterior horn inserts into the fossa intercondylaris femoris and via a strong fasciculus that proceeds upward and medially. This is known as the ligament of Wrisberg and often blends with the posterior cruciate ligament.

The lateral meniscus has very loose connections to the lateral capsule and its posterior horn has the popliteus tendon sheath interposed between it and the capsule. A synovial pouch (recessus inferior) may occur between the meniscus and the capsule. Its outer wall contains the popliteus tendon; this compartment is called the sheath of the popliteus tendon. The lateral meniscus has great mobility because of its bony connection centrally with the spines and little or no lateral capsular connection.

5

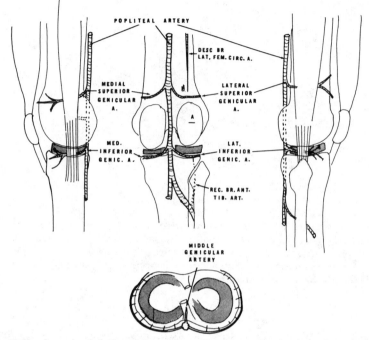

FIGURE 5. Blood supply of the knee joint. The popliteal artery has five branches in the area of the knee joint.

BLOOD SUPPLY

The popliteal artery, a continuation of the femoral artery, has five branches in the area of the knee joint (Fig. 5): the medial and lateral superior geniculars, the middle genicular, and the medial and lateral inferior geniculars.

The superior geniculars curve around the femoral condyles proximal to the epicondyles and form a plexus in the suprapatellar area. The inferior genicular branches course around the margin of the tibial plateau passing under the collateral ligaments. The middle genicular arises from the posterior portion of the popliteal artery, pierces the popliteal ligament, and sends three branches: the middle follows the anterior cruciate ligament and the medial and lateral branches enter the perimeniscal connective tissue zone (Fig. 6).

The middle and inferior genicular branches supply the menisci, which are mostly avascular. Only the outer one third and the central portion of the meniscus have any significant blood supply.

The superior genicular plexus is joined by the descending branch of the lateral femoral circumflex artery and the inferior genicular plexus is joined by the recurrent branch of the anterior tibial artery.

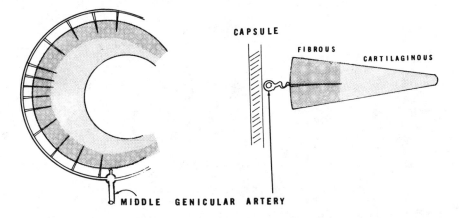

CAPSULE

FIBROUS

CARTILAGINOUS

MIDDLE GENICULAR ARTERY

FIGURE 6. Intrinsic circulation of the menisci. The middle genicular artery sends branches around the loose connective tissue of the perimeniscal zone under the capsule. Nonanastomatic small vessels, tortuous to permit movement, enter the fibrous zone (outer third) of the meniscus. They are more numerous in the central area of the meniscus. The inner third (cartilaginous zone) is avascular.

LIGAMENTS

The bony configuration of the knee joint contributes little to the stability and integrity of the joint. Strength is dependent upon the integrity of the muscles and secondarily upon the ligaments. The ligaments comprising the joint structure are the cruciates, the collaterals, and the joint capsule.

Cruciate

The paired cruciate ligaments are named according to their tibial attachments. The anterior cruciate ligament proceeds superiorly and posteriorly from its anterior medial tibial attachment to attach to the medial aspect of the lateral femoral condyle (Fig. 7) and the posterior cruciate arises from the back of the tibia and extends forward, upward, and inward to attach to the medial femoral condyle. The cruciate ligaments prevent shear motion of the knee joint and act to guide the flexion-rotation of the knee joint. The posterior cruciate ligament prevents excessive *internal* rotation of the tibia upon the femur. The anterior cruciate prevents abnormal *external* rotation.

By its attachment and direction (Fig. 8), the anterior cruciate ligament stabilizes the knee in extension and prevents hyperextension. The posterior cruciate aids normal knee flexion by acting as a drag during the primary glide.

7

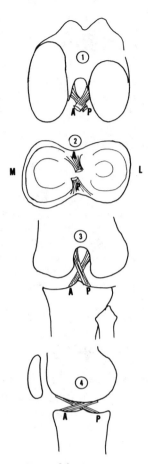

FIGURE 7. Cruciate ligaments. *1*, Viewed from posterior aspect of right knee with knee bent; *2*, Superior view of tibial plateau; *3*, Posterior view of extended right knee; *4*, Side view of knee.

A = Anterior ligaments
P = Posterior ligaments
M = Medial ligaments
L = Lateral ligaments

Capsular and Collateral

The capsular and collateral ligaments stabilize the joint by guiding, as well as restricting joint motion. The collateral ligaments are essentially a selective thickening of the fibrous capsule of the joint. They can be divided into medial and lateral portions, each having specific characteristics (Fig. 9).

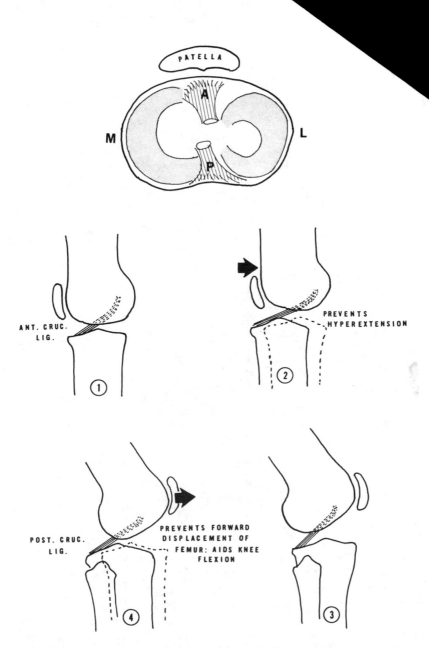

Figure 8. Function and restriction imposed upon cruciate ligaments. *Top*, Superior view of the point of attachment and direction of the cruciates. Right knee medial aspect: *1*, Direction of anterior cruciate and (*2*) method of preventing hyperextension of the knee. Right knee lateral aspect: *3*, The posterior cruciate ligament and (*4*) manner in which it prevents forward displacement of the femur upon the tibia. By acting as a drag force it aids in normal knee flexion.

9

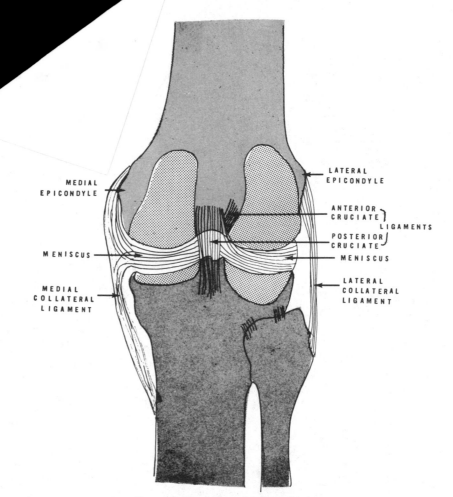

MEDIAL
EPICONDYLE

LATERAL
EPICONDYLE

ANTERIOR
CRUCIATE ⎤
⎦ LIGAMENTS
POSTERIOR ⎰
CRUCIATE ⎱

MENISCUS

MENISCUS

MEDIAL
COLLATERAL
LIGAMENT

LATERAL
COLLATERAL
LIGAMENT

FIGURE 9. Capsular and collateral ligaments.

MEDIAL PORTION. The medial capsular ligaments divide into deep and superficial sections. The *deep section* in turn is divisable into three portions: the anterior, middle, and posterior ligaments (Fig. 10). The anterior portion has parallel fibers that cover the anterior aspect of the joint, extend anteriorly into the extension mechanism, and attach loosely to the medial meniscus. These fibers are slightly relaxed during knee extension but become taut during flexion (Fig. 11). The posterior fibers are oblique (fanned), thin, and indistinct. They continue posteriorly to aid in the formation of the posterior popliteal capsule. They are attached to the posterior medial aspect of the medial meniscus and blend with the semimembranosus muscle. The middle third of the deep medial capsular ligament has more distinct fibers and comprises a superior and inferior divi-

10

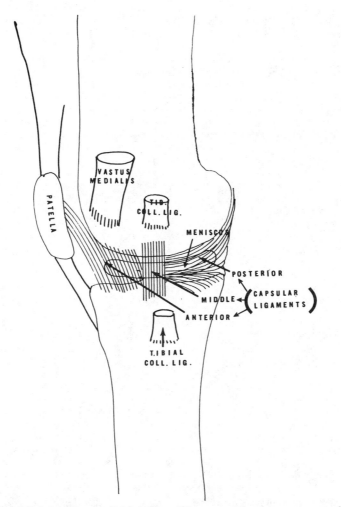

FIGURE 10. Medial (tibial) superficial collateral ligament. The three segments of the deep medial capsular ligament are shown: the parallel fibers of the anterior portion, the middle vertical, and the fanned indistinct posterior fibers. The superficial collateral ligament attaches just superior to the femoral medial epicondyle and to the tibia just below the articular cartilage and posterior to a point above the insertion of the semimembranous tendon.

sion (Fig. 12). The superior (meniscofemoral segment) is thicker and fixes the medial meniscus to the femur, the inferior (meniscotibial) is looser and permits the tibia to move upon the meniscus.

The medial collateral ligament is principally the *superficial section* of the medial ligament. It attaches superiorly to the femoral medial epicondyle and inferiorly upon the tibia just below the level of the articular cartilage. The anterior fibers are parallel and distinct. The posterior fibers converge into oblique fibers that are thinner and less distinct and

11

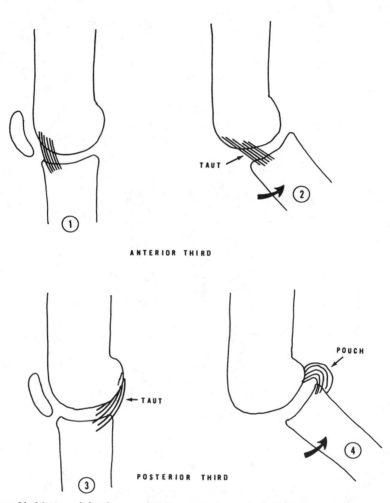

ANTERIOR THIRD

POSTERIOR THIRD

FIGURE 11. Motion of the deep medial ligaments during knee flexion. *1*, The anterior fibers are slightly slack during knee extension and *(2)* taut during flexion. *3 and 4*, The opposite action of the posterior fibers.

that blend into the deep posterior capsular ligaments and into the semi-membranous muscle tendon. Fibers from the posterior fibers attach to the medial meniscus. Numerous bursa (usually five) are interposed between the deep middle capsular ligament and the superficial collateral ligament (see Fig. 12).

LATERAL PORTION. The fibular collateral ligament passes from the lateral epicondyle of the femur to the head of the fibula (Fig. 13) where it is surrounded by the divided tendons of the biceps. The popliteus tendon passes beneath the fibular (lateral) ligament as it passes to attach to the lateral epicondyle of the femur. The underlying capsule thickens in its

12

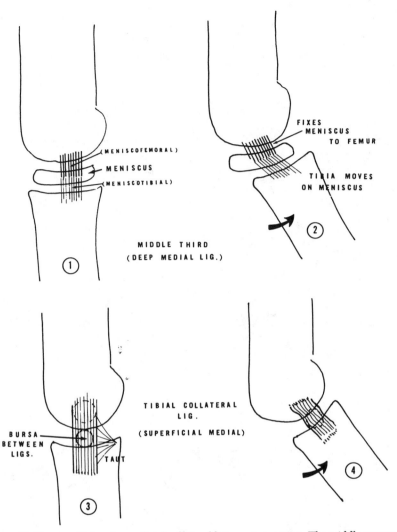

FIGURE 12. Deep medial and superficial collateral ligamentous action. The middle segment of the deep medial capsular ligament is divided into (1) a superior portion that fixes the medial meniscus to the femur during flexion and (2) an inferior portion that is slack and permits the meniscus to move. Joint spaces called meniscofemoral and meniscotibial are arbitrarily formed. 3 and 4 show the relationship of a bursa to the superficial and deep medial liagments.

extension from the lateral femoral condyle to the fibular head to form a short fibular collateral ligament called the arcuate ligament.

The posterior border of the arcuate lies over the popliteal fascia, covering it and attached firmly to it. The arcuate is also firmly attached to the posterior arch of the lateral meniscus. The upper fibers of the popliteus muscle attach to the arcuate ligament and the lateral meniscus (see Fig.

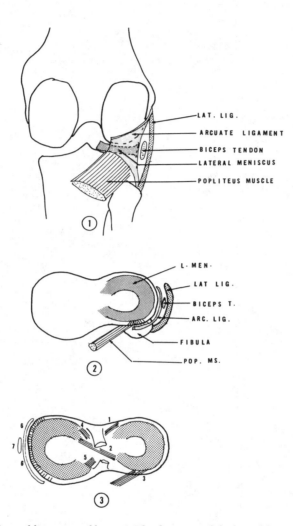

FIGURE 13. Lateral ligaments of knee. *1,* The deep part of the lateral ligament attaches from the femoral epicondyle to the styloid process and tibial border of the fibular head. The posterior border lying across the popliteus muscle forms the arcuate ligament. The arcuate ligament attaches firmly to the posterior horn of the lateral ligament. Between the lateral ligament attachment and the arcuate ligament passes the tendon of the biceps femoris muscle. *2,* The popliteus muscle emerges beneath the arcuate ligament to insert medioposteriorly on the tibia. The muscle originates partly from the arcuate ligament margin and from the posterior aspect of the meniscus. When the knee flexes, this muscle probably pulls the meniscus and simultaneously externally rotates itself, thus protecting the meniscus. *3,* Attachment of menisci. The lateral menisci is attached at both horns to the tibia *(1-2)* with *2* crossing over from the posterior horn of the lateral meniscus to the anterior horn of the medial meniscus and the femoral attachment of the anterior cruciate ligament. There are fibrous bands *(1-4)* that connect anterior horns of both menisci to the femoral attachments of the anterior cruciate. The medial meniscus is attached by its anterior and posterior horns with fibrous bands *4-5,* and along the entire circumference of the capsule *(6)* and the superficial medial ligament *(7).*

14

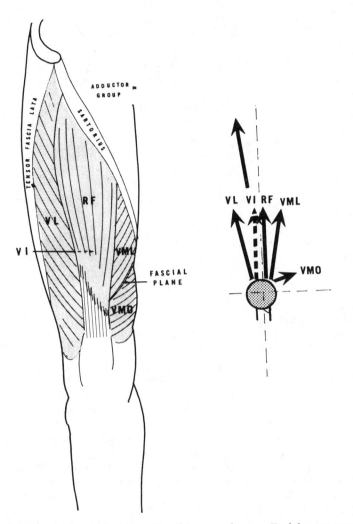

FIGURE 14. Quadriceps femoris: function of quadriceps mechanism. Each long component of the quadriceps group (*RF*, rectus femoris; *VL*, vastus lateralis; *VI*, vastus intermedius; *VM*, vastus medialis) can extend the knee fully. The vastus medialis oblique fibers *(VMO)* cannot extend the knee but apparently pull the patella medially (right) and keep it centered against lateral pull of the quadriceps *(arrows)*. All long components pull equally throughout extension range with *VMO* exerting twice the force of contraction. The mechanics of the joint determine weakness (less efficiency) in the last 15 to 20°.

13). The peroneal nerve passes the neck of the fibula behind the biceps tendon.

The posterior popliteal fossa of the knee joint is bounded superiorly by the semimembranosus and semitendinosus tendons and the biceps tendon and inferiorly by the two heads of the gastrocnemius muscle. The roof

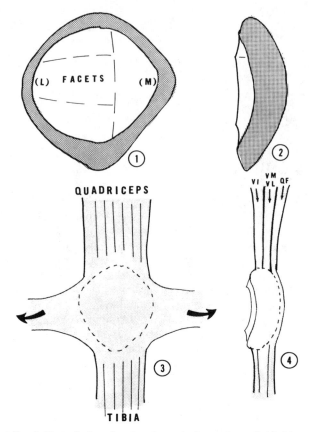

FIGURE 15. Patella. *1*, Ventral view showing the articular surfaces divided into three medial facets and a lateral facet that articulate with the femur. The lateral aspect is wider than the medial. The rough bone presents the surface upon which the patellar extensor mechanism attaches. *2*, Lateral view of the patella. *3*, The quadriceps attaches to the patella. Laterally and medially *(arrows)*, fibers extend to attach to the femoral condyles and the capsulomeniscal tissues. *4*, The three layers of the tendinous insertion. The quadriceps *(QR)* covers the anterior aspect of the patella. The vasti medialis and lateralis *(VM and VL)* attach to the middle (superior and lateral) aspects of the patella and the vastus intermedius *(VI)* to the posterior (superior) margin.

consists of the popliteal fascia under which lie the popliteal artery, vein, and nerve. The popliteal nerve divides into the tibial and peroneal branches in the upper portion of the fossa with the peroneal branch passing over the lateral head of the gastrocnemius under the fascia.

MUSCLES

The knee is powerfully motored and stabilized by muscles that cross the joint from origin above the hip joint, from the entire femoral shaft, and

16

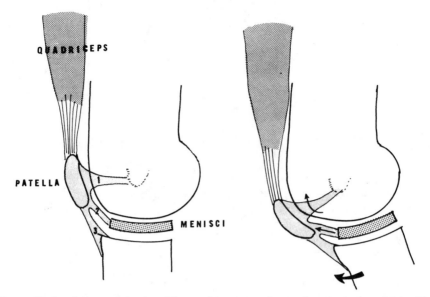

FIGURE 16. Quadriceps mechanism. The quadriceps extends over the anterior knee joint with three ligamentous extensions: *1*, the epicondylopatellar portion attaches to the epicondyle eminence of the femur and guides rotation of the patella; *2*, the meniscopatellar attaches to and pulls the meniscus forward during knee extension; and *3*, the infrapatellar tendon, which attaches to the tibial tubercle and extends the tibia upon the femur.

from origin above the knee of lower leg muscles. For convenience, muscle groups can be classified as anterior (knee *extensor*), posterior, (knee *flexors*), medial (*adductors*), and lateral (*abductors*). Both abductors and adductors are also rotators and stabilizers.

Anterior

The major muscle of the extensor group is the quadriceps femoris, comprising four heads: the rectus femoris and three vasti named the medialis, lateralis, and intermedius. The rectus originates from the anterior inferior iliac spine; thus, it crosses the hip joint and influences hip motion. The vasti arise from the shaft of the femur. All four muscles converge into a common tendon that crosses the knee joint and attaches to the tibial tuberosity (Fig. 14) via the patella.

The patella (Fig. 15), long considered a sesamoid bone, provides with the femur, a gliding surface that minimizes frictional attrition and provides mechanical leverage (Figs. 16 and 17). The quadriceps femoris tendon comprises three lamina: the superficial layer from the rectus, the middle layer from tendons of the vasti lateralis and medialis, and a deep layer from the vastus intermedius. Some of the tendon fibers pass over (anterior to) the patella; some attach to the superior and some to the

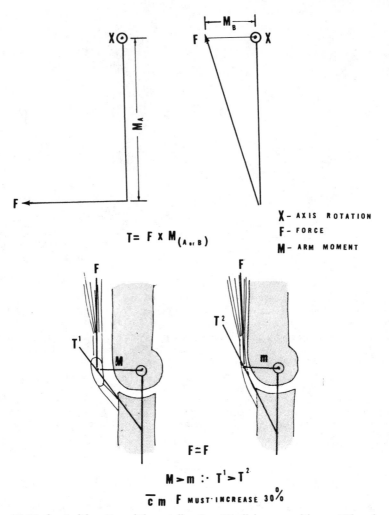

$$T = F \times M_{(A \text{ or } B)}$$

X – AXIS ROTATION
F – FORCE
M – ARM MOMENT

F = F

$$M > m \therefore T^1 > T^2$$

c m F MUST INCREASE 30%

FIGURE 17. Mechanical function of the patella. *Top*, Parallelograms of forces. When force is applied perpendicular to arm to rotate around axis *(X)*, torque *(T)* equals force *(F)* times length of arm (M_A). With force applied oblique to arm, the moment becomes the distance from the force to the axis; thus $T = F \times M_B$. *Bottom*, In the knee, the patella increases the arm moment from *m* to *M* and thus torque T^1 is greater than T^2 with similar force *(F)*. If the patella is not present, it has been calculated that a 30 percent increase in quadriceps strength is necessary to create equal torque. These forces are computed to knee rotation but disregard translation (gliding).

lateral borders of the patella. Fibers from the lateral and medial aspects of the patella fan out to either side to insert into the femoral condyles (see Fig. 15) and some fibers pass to the capsular and collateral ligaments to attach to the menisci (see Fig. 16).

Superficial to the quadriceps in the anterior aspect of the thigh is the sartorius muscle. This ribbonlike muscle spirals across the thigh from its

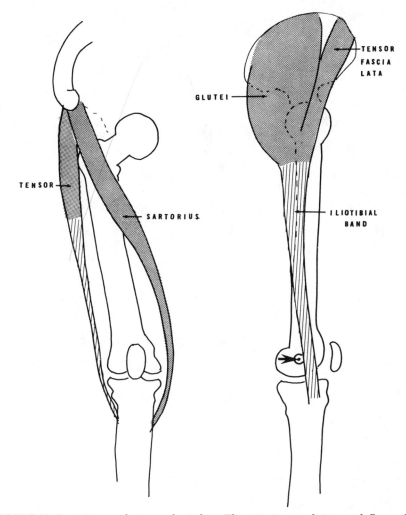

FIGURE 18. Sartorius muscle: tensor fascia lata. The sartorius muscle is a weak flexor of the knee and hip. The tensor fascia lata, which acts upon the knee, is considered to be a knee extensor but its primary function is abduction and stabilization of the hip.

origin at the anterosuperior spine to the anterosuperior-medial portion of the tibia (Fig. 18). Although there are other thigh muscles (the lateral and medial groups: the adductors and abductors), they function mostly upon the hip joint and will not be detailed here. Reference to standard texts is encouraged.

The nerve supply of the quadriceps group is the femoral nerve, which is formed by the anterior primary division of L_{2-4}. Its sensory distribution is depicted in Figure 19. In addition to motor function, the knee-jerk (deep tendon) reflex is dependent upon the integrity of this nerve and its roots.

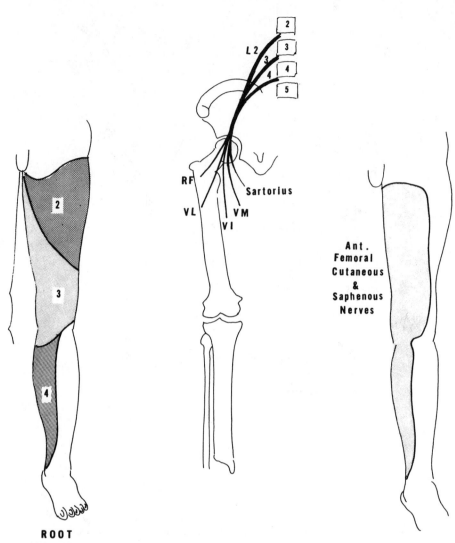

ROOT DERMATOMES

FIGURE 19. Distribution of the femoral nerve: its root formation. *Left,* Root dermatomes of the leg and thigh. *Center,* Formation of the nerve with anterior primary divisions of L_2, L_3, and L_4. *Right,* Cutaneous sensory distribution of the lower extremity.

Posterior

The posterior thigh and leg muscles also cross the knee and act to flex and rotate the leg upon the femur. They can best be divided into the medial and lateral groups (Fig. 20). The medial group contains the semi-membranosus and semitendinosus muscles, which, when the knee is

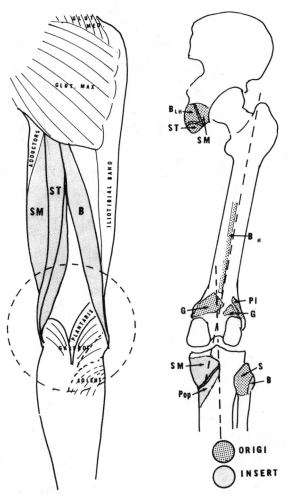

Figure 20. Posterior thigh muscles: flexors. *Left,* The semimembranosus *(SM);* semitendinosus *(ST),* and the biceps femoris *(B).* The other muscles are labelled. *Right,* The origin and insertion of the posterior muscle groups.

B_{LH} = Biceps long head
B_{SH} = Biceps short head
B = Biceps
S = Sartorius
Pl = Plantaris
Pop = Popliteus
G = Heads of gastrocnemius

flexed, internally rotate the lower leg upon the femur. The biceps femoris is the main lateral muscle of the hamstring group and, when the knee is flexed, it rotates the leg externally (Fig. 21).

The semitendinosus muscle originates from the ischial tuberosity (see Fig. 20), blending with the origin of the long head of the biceps femoris.

21

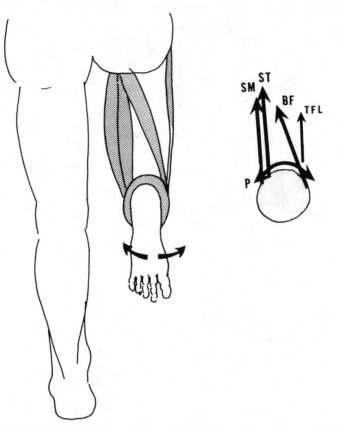

FIGURE 21. Rotators of the leg. When the knee is flexed the semimembranosus *(SM)* and the semitendinosus *(ST)* inwardly rotate the tibia. The biceps femoris *(BF)* and the tensor fascia lata *(TFL)* externally rotate the leg. The popliteus *(P)* originating laterally and inserting medially, internally rotates the leg upon the femur.

After descending the medial aspect of the thigh, it crosses the knee joint and joins the sartorius and gracilis muscles in a tendon, the pes anserinus, which flexes the knee (Fig. 22).

The semimembranosus arises from the ischial tuberosity lateral to the semitendinosus and descends the femur under the semitendinosus. It inserts by four tendons into the posteromedial side of the medial tibial condyle (Fig. 23) and sends fibers anteriorly to blend into the medial capsule and posteriorly to blend with the popliteal capsule. A deep fibrous branching attaches to the posterior horn of the medial meniscus and pulls the meniscus posteriorly when the semimembranosus flexes the knee.

The lateral flexor of the knee is primarily the biceps femoris muscle. The long head originates in the ischial tuberosity, descends the posterior thigh, and merges with the short head that originates from the linea aspera of the femur. The long head forms a broad flat tendon 7 to 10 cm

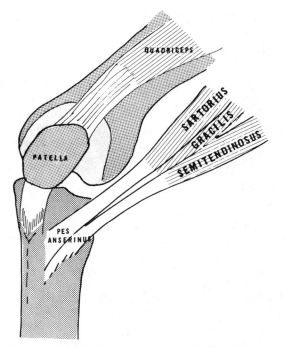

FIGURE 22. Pes anserinus. The medial insertion of the outer hamstring group forms a conjoined tendon of the semitendinosus with the sartorius and the gracilis muscles to form the pes anserinus. This tendon is separated from the underlying femoral condyle by a bursa.

above the level of the knee joint. It is joined on its undersurface at the fibular head to form a thick common tendon (Fig. 24).

The common biceps tendon passes downward and forward toward the knee joint. When it reaches the collateral ligament it splits into three layers: the superficial, middle, and deep.

The *superficial layer* forms three expansions: an anterior, middle, and posterior expansion. The anterior (Fig. 25) is thin, but strong, and fans out forward and down the lower leg. The middle expansion is thin and splits to surround the collateral ligament; these expansion layers are separated from the ligament by bursae medially (inner), anteriorly, and laterally (outer). The posterior expansion is connected to the collateral ligament and to the joint capsule by a firm fibrous attachment. The *deep layer* bifurcates into a fibular and a tibial attachment (see Fig. 25) passing behind (medial to) the collateral ligament before attaching into the fibular head and the posterior aspect of the joint capsule.

The biceps femoris muscle functions to flex and to rotate externally the leg upon the femur when the knee is flexed (see Fig. 21). Passively pulling the superficial layer of the biceps insertion tendon flexes the knee and externally rotates the leg. As the knee flexes, the *middle layer* pulls upon

23

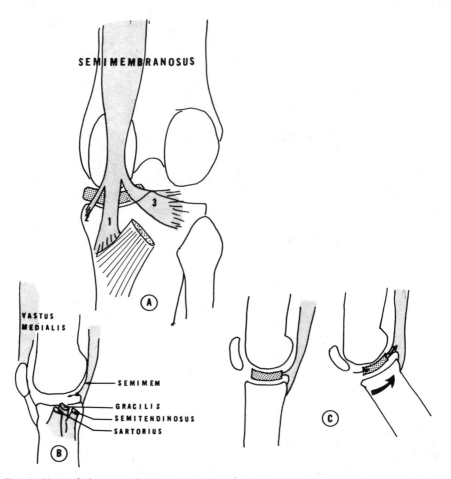

FIGURE 23. Medial aspect of the posterior knee structure. *A,* The semimembranosus muscle has four tendinous inserts. The major insert *(1)* extends to attach on the posterior aspect of the tibia and sends fibers into the popliteus. In its path there is an exterior branch that attaches to the posterior aspect of the medial meniscus *(2 and 3).* These tendons complete the posterior popliteal fossa and tense the capsule. *B,* The medial aspect of the knee with the insertion sites of the medial flexors. *C,* The semimembranosus flexes the knee and simultaneously pulls the meniscus backward and rotates it with the tibia.

the collateral ligament causing it to bow posteriorly and causing some slack in it. By its attachment of the deep portion to the joint capsule, as the knee flexes this middle layer expansion prevents impingement of the capsule between the tibia and the femur. This expansion is also attached to the tensor (iliotibial band) and thus keeps the iliotibial band taut through knee flexion. As the biceps tendon middle layer bows the collateral ligament to maintain slack, it tightens the iliotibial band; this latter is most taut at 10 to 30° of flexion.

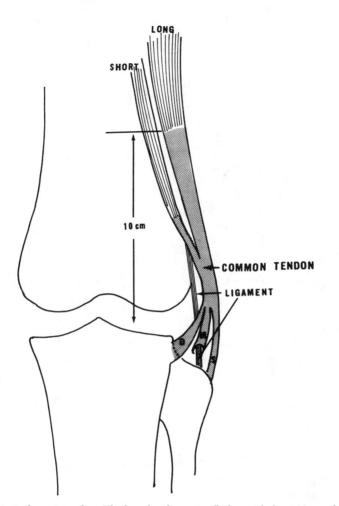

FIGURE 24. Biceps femoris tendon. The long head remains fleshy until about 10 cm above the knee joint where it becomes a flat tendon. The short head remains fleshy until the fibular head. The common tendon then splits into three layers: superficial (S), middle (M), and deep (D).

The flexor muscles receive their nerve supply from the sciatic nerve. After the sciatic nerve divides into its tibial and common peroneal nerve, the tibial nerve supplies the semimembranosus, semitendinosus, and the long head of the biceps; the short head of the biceps is supplied by the common peroneal branch.

The popliteus muscle forms a part of the floor of the posterior knee fossa. It arises from the lateral epicondyle of the femur and runs postero-medially to attach to the posterior surface of the tibia. It rotates the leg internally upon the femur and is a weak knee flexor.

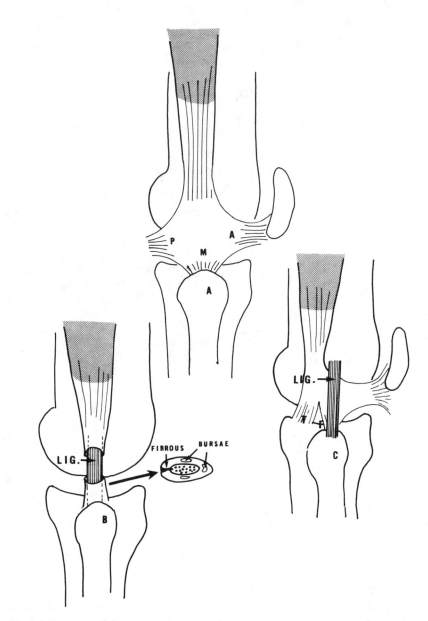

FIGURE 25. Layers of the common biceps tendon. *A,* Superficial layer. The tendon divides into three expansions: anterior *(A)*, which fans out to blend with the anterior crural fascia; middle *(M)*, which extends to the collateral ligament at the fibular head; posterior *(P)*, which blends with the fascia of the calf and lateral leg muscles. *B,* Middle layer. This is a thin layer that splits to envelop the lateral collateral ligament. The insert depicts the relationship of the bursae and the posterior fibrous attachment to the ligament. *C,* Deep layer. This layer bifurcates with one portion attaching to the fibular head *(F)* and the anterior half passing behind (medial to) the ligament and attaching to the tibia *(T)*. Both attach to the knee joint capsule.

26

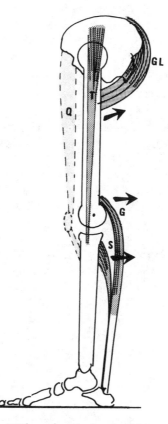

Figure 26. Standing balance. With nonfunctioning quadriceps, stance is possible by ligamentous support (the posterior popliteal capsule and anterior [hip joint capsule] Y ligament of Bigelow) and by gastrocnemius action. In the weight-bearing position, the gastrocnemius can be considered to originate from the calcaneus and insert the upper tibia and distal femur, thus extending the knee.

Gastrocnemius

The gastrocnemius muscles, essentially plantar flexors of the foot and ankle, by their origin above the knee joint have an effect on the knee joint. The gastrocnemius arises from two heads, medial and lateral, from the epicondyles of the femur. They quickly unite and descend the leg, joining the soleus muscle below the knee joint. The conjoined tendon ultimately attaches to the calcaneus.

When the leg is not weight bearing, the gastrocnemius acts to flex the knee; when it is weight bearing, the gastrocnemius *extends* the knee (Fig. 26). Without the quadriceps functioning, the leg can be fully extended and can become a stable weight-bearing extremity. The foot, fixed to the

27

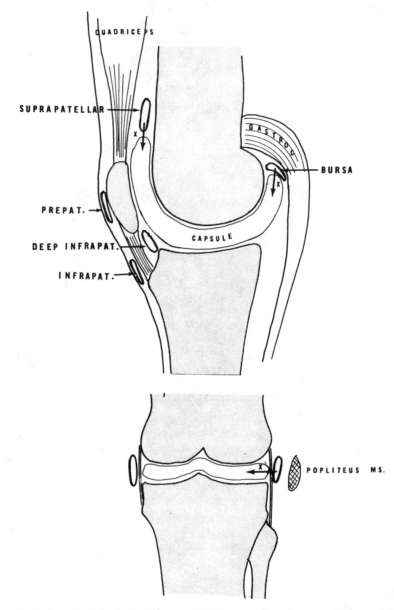

FIGURE 27. Bursae about the knee. Bursae noted: *Suprapatellar,* also termed the quadriceps femoral bursa, may communicate with the knee capsule; *Prepatellar,* between the skin and patella; *Infrapatellar* (superficial), between the skin and infrapatellar ligament; *Deep Infrapatellar,* between infrapatellar ligament and tibia; and bursae between the lateral head of the gastrocnemius and the joint capsule, the fibular collateral ligament and the biceps or popliteal tendon, and the popliteal tendon and the lateral femoral condyle. X indicates possible communication with the joint capsule.

floor, becomes the *origin* of the gastrocnemius that now can be considered to *insert* to the lower femur and upper tibia and pull these posteriorly, thus extending the knee. The knee joint now *locks* on its posterior capsule. At the hip joint, the gluteus maximus extends the femur and weight bearing is now borne upon the anterior (hip joint capsule) Y ligament of Bigelow. Erect stance is now accomplished by ligamentous structures and minimal sporadic isometric contractions of the gastrocnemius and soleus muscles.

BURSAE

Bursae are normally located at sites of moving tissue to permit friction-free action and diminish attrition and inflammation of these contiguous tissues. There are 11 or more bursae in the region of the knee joint (Fig. 27). Three communicate with the knee joint: quadriceps (suprapatellar), popliteus, and the medial gastrocnemius. Three are related to the patella and the patellar tendon: prepatellar, superficial infrapatellar, and the deep infrapatellar. Two relate to the semimembranosus tendons: one, which communicates with the gastrocnemius bursa or the knee joint, or both, lies between the semimembranosus tendons and the gastrocnemius tendon, and the other lies between the semimembranosus tendon and the tibial condyle.

Two bursae lie superficially to the collateral ligaments: one between the fibular collateral ligament and the overlying biceps tendon and the other between the tibial collateral ligament and the three overlying tendons of the pes anserinus (the sartorius, gracilis, and semitendinosus). One bursa exists between the superficial and the deep parts of the tibial collateral ligaments. Irritation, inflammation, and infection of these bursae must be considered in the differential diagnosis of knee pain (see Chapter 6).

A pain in the posterior knee frequently can present itself; its causation and exact area are not always clear. This is the so-called Baker's cyst. Numerous posterior bursal inflammations are so termed. These may include bursitis between the medial head of the gastrocnemius and the semimembranosus tendon, which may communicate with the capsule space; a synovial cyst of the semitendinosus tendon; or more important may resemble a cyst and instead be an aneurysm of the popliteal artery, an A-V fistula, or a soft tissue tumor. Proper diagnosis frequently is followed by exploratory or curative surgery.

BIBLIOGRAPHY

BASMAJIAN, JV: *Grant's Method of Anatomy.* Williams & Wilkins, Baltimore, 1971.

BASMAJIAN, JV AND LOVEJOY, JF: *Function of the popliteus muscle in man.* J Bone Joint Surg 53-A:557, 1971.

BRANTIGAN, OC AND VOSHELL, AF: *Tibial collateral ligament: Its function, its bursae, and its relation to the medial meniscus.* J Bone Joint Surg 25:1, 1943.

DEPALMA, AF: *Diseases of the Knee: Management and Surgery.* JB Lippincott, Philadelphia, 1954.

HELFET, AJ: *Mechanism of derangements of the medial semilunar cartilage and their management.* J Bone Joint Surg 41-B:319, 1959.

HELFET, AJ: *Function of cruciate ligaments of knee-joint.* Lancet 1:665, 1948.

LAST, RJ: *Some anatomical details of the knee joint.* J Bone Joint Surg 30-B:683, 1948.

LIEB, FJ AND PERRY, J: *Quadriceps function. An electromyographic study under isometric conditions.* J Bone Joint Surg 53-A:749, 1971.

MARSHAL, JL, GIRGIS, FG, AND ZELKO, RR: *The biceps femoris tendon and its functional significance.* J Bone Joint Surg 54-A:1444,1972.

REIDEK, B, ET AL: *The anterior aspect of the knee joint: An anatomical study.* J Bone Joint Surg 63-A:351, 1981.

RICKLIN, P, RUTTMANN, A, AND DEL BUONO, MS: *Meniscus Lesions: Practical Problems of Clinical Diagnosis, Arthrography, and Therapy.* Grune & Stratton, New York, 1971.

SEEBACHER, JR, ET AL: *The structure of the posterolateral aspect of the knee.* J Bone Joint Surg 64-A:536, 1982.

SLOCUM, DB, AND LARSON, RL: *Rotatory instability of the knee.* J Bone Joint Surg 50-A:211, 1968.

THOREK, SL: *Orthopaedics: Principles and Their Application,* ed 2. JB Lippincott, Philadelphia, 1967.

WARREN, LF AND MARSHALL, JL: *The supporting structures and layers of the medial side of the knee: An anatomical analysis.* J Bone Joint Surg 61-A:56, 1979.

CHAPTER 2

Functional Anatomy

Knee flexion or extension is accompanied by a gliding motion of the tibia upon the femur with simultaneous rotation. There is external rotation of the tibia upon the femur during knee extension and internal rotation during flexion. The first 20° of flexion causes a rocking motion. After 20°, further flexion is composed of a gliding motion (Fig. 28).

After 20° of flexion the ligaments become relaxed and permit both gliding and axial rotation. Most rotation occurs during the final phase of full flexion and during the last 30 to 40° of extension. Some rotation, however, occurs throughout the entire flexion and extension action (Fig. 29). At 90° of knee flexion, 30 to 40° of rotation of the tibia upon the femur is possible. In full extension *no* axial rotation is possible (Fig. 29). The anterior fibers of the tibial collateral ligaments incline forward as they descend to insert upon the tibia. This obliquely blocks rotation of the tibia (Fig. 30). As the knee flexes, the superficial collateral ligament moves posterior and becomes slack, thus permitting rotation (see Fig. 30). The deep capsular ligament becomes taut and is left to resist excessive rotation.

As the tibia rotates upon the femur, the capsule tightens and further compresses the femoral and tibial articular surfaces together. Further rotation past its physiologic limits tears the capsule. In full knee extension *no* significant medial or lateral abduction of the tibia upon the femur is permitted. The anterior cruciate ligament *unwinds* during the first 15 to 20° external rotation. As further outward rotation occurs, the anterior cruciate ligament becomes more taut as it winds around the medial aspect of the lateral femoral condyle (Fig. 31).

The posterior third of the medial meniscus blocks external rotation of the tibia upon the femur. The vastus medialis inhibits outward rotation of the tibia during the first 60° of flexion of the knee. The vastus medialis originates from the intermuscular system and the medial epicondyle of the femur and extends downward and laterally to extend into the extensor

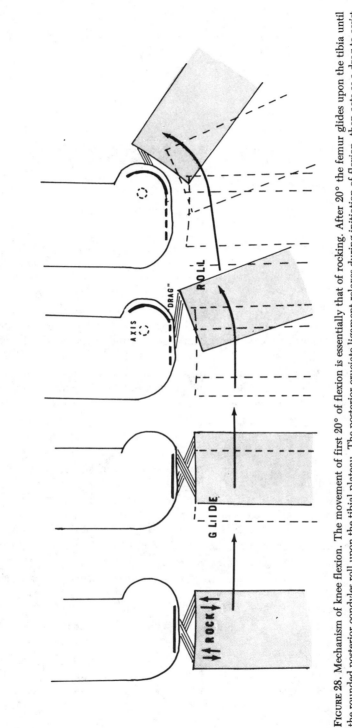

FIGURE 28. Mechanism of knee flexion. The movement of first 20° of flexion is essentially that of rocking. After 20° the femur glides upon the tibia until the rounded posterior condyles roll upon the tibial plateau. The posterior cruciate ligament relaxes during initiation of flexion, then acts as a drag to assist further flexion.

32

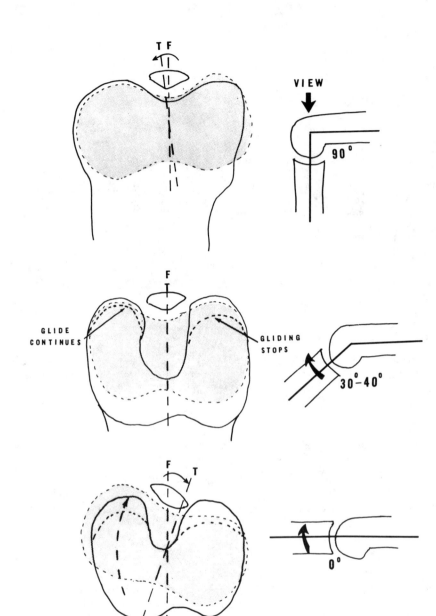

RIGHT KNEE

FIGURE 29. Functional evaluation of knee flexion-extension. With knee flexed to 90°, 40° of rotation is possible. Active flexion has simultaneous internal rotation. In full extension the tibia is externally rotated upon the femur.

33

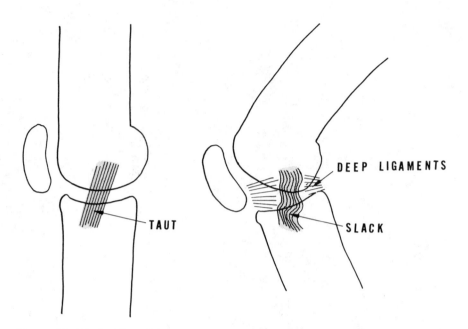

FIGURE 30. Tibial collateral ligament. *Left,* Fully extended knee, the superficial medial ligament is oblique to alignment of leg and prevents axial roation. *Right,* Knee is flexed causing ligament to become slack and allowing tibia to rotate. The deep medial ligament becomes taut and restricts rotation.

aponeurosis and the patella. When the vastus medialis contracts, it moves the patella medially and upward (Fig. 32).

Rotation of the tibia upon the femur during flexion-extension is passive because of the anatomic configuration of the articular surfaces. The muscles acting upon the joint all have a rotatory torque action but this is secondary. During flexion-extension, the tibia follows the configuration of the medial condyle of the femur, which is longer than the lateral condyle (Fig. 33).

As the femur glides upon the tibia, it stops when the surface contour of the lateral condyle has been traversed but continues to move along the longer and more curved medial condyle, which curves in a lateral direction. During extension, the tibia rotates upon the femur a distance equal to half the width of the patella (Fig. 34). The knee extensors (quadriceps) run medially and thus help rotate the tibia during extension (see Fig. 14).

Flexion from the fully extended position begins with simultaneous internal rotation (tibia upon the femur) by contraction of the popliteus muscle. Further active flexion results from hamstring contraction. The capsular ligaments, which are taut during full extension, relax as flexion begins. The femur glides forward upon the tibia (see Fig. 33), placing the

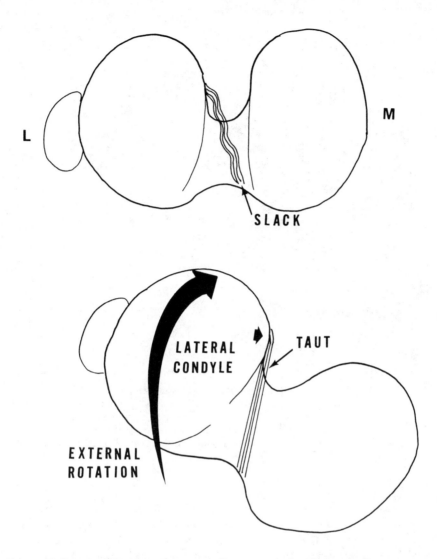

L

M

SLACK

LATERAL
CONDYLE

TAUT

EXTERNAL
ROTATION

FIGURE 31. Rotational limitation by cruciate ligaments. As the tibia externally rotates upon the femur, the cruciate ligament becomes slack. As rotation progresses, the anterior cruciate wraps around the medial aspect of the lateral femoral condyle to become taut and restrict further rotation.

smaller rounded posterior surface of the femoral condyles upon the tibial plateau.

The posterior cruciate ligament becomes taut (see Fig. 8) and acts as a drag to any further forward gliding. An axis now exists around which the tibia rotates upon the femur.

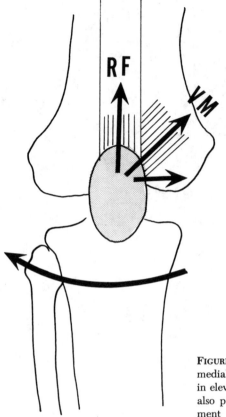

FIGURE 32. Vastus medialis function. The vastus medialis *(VM)* assists the quadriceps femoris *(RF)* in elevating the patella and extending the knee. It also pulls the patella medially to align its movement and limits external rotation of the tibia *(curved arrow)*.

In flexion and extension, the menisci, fixed to the tibia, move with it upon the femur. In rotation, with the knee flexed, the menisci move with the femur upon the tibia. If the femoral-meniscotibial spaces are considered to be joint spaces the upper femoral-meniscal joint moves during flexion-extension and rotation occurs at the lower meniscotibial joint (see Fig. 12).

The menisci have firm ligamentous attachments. The medial meniscus is attached at both horns and along its entire outer circumferential border. The lateral meniscus is attached at both horns but the remainder of its lateral (outer) margin is free.

The cruciate ligaments crisscross. The anterior cruciate is taut during extension and unwinds and relaxes during flexion. The collateral ligaments, also taut during extension, relax during flexion—the lateral more than the medial (Fig. 35). As ligamentous relaxation occurs during flex-

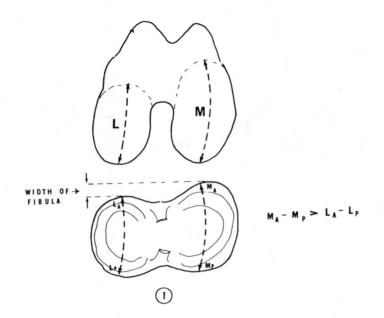

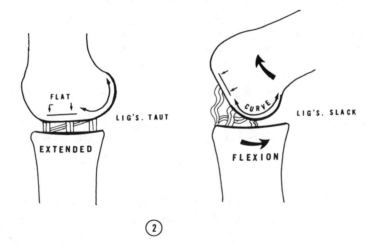

$$M_A - M_P > L_A - L_P$$

FIGURE 33. Passive mechanism of flexion-extension. *1*, The lateral condyle of the femur, L_A-L_P, is shorter than the medial condyle, M_A-M_P, thus the femur travels further on the medial surface as the quadriceps muscle continues to contract when the lateral motion ceases. Motion continues about half an inch and the femur continues to move upon the tibia, causing the tibia to rotate externally (outward). *2*, The knee is stable in full extension. The flat anterior surface of the femoral condyles fit into the tibial condyles and the ligaments are taut. The tibial intercondylar eminences prevent lateral gliding.

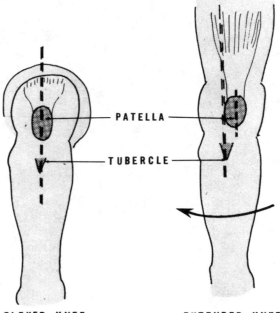

PATELLA

TUBERCLE

FLEXED KNEE   EXTENDED KNEE

FIGURE 34. Surface manifestation of tibial rotation. When the flexed knee is viewed from the front, the patella lies directly over the tibial tubercle. With the knee fully extended the tubercle is lateral to the patella, indicating external rotation during knee extension.

ion, some axial rotation is permitted and the axis of rotation moves posteriorly (Fig. 36).

The external rotation of the tibia upon the femur during the last 20° of extension is termed the "screw home" mechanism and, as stated, is due to condylar configuration, muscle torque action, and ligamentous guidance.

When the knee extends because of contraction of the quadriceps, the patella is forcefully pulled upward. The infrapatellar fat pad and the alar ligaments connected to the joint capsule are also pulled anterior and upward, thus preventing their being impinged between the opposing condyles. The three facets on the dorsal surface of the patella simultaneously alternate their contact with the femoral patellar surface. From flexion to extension the contact goes from superior facet to middle to inferior.

Muscular action in extension is essentially that of the quadriceps femoris group. The rectus femoris alone cannot fully extend the leg; the vasti, especially the vastus medialis, perform this function. The patella mechanically increases the efficacy of the extensor mechanism by improving leverage.

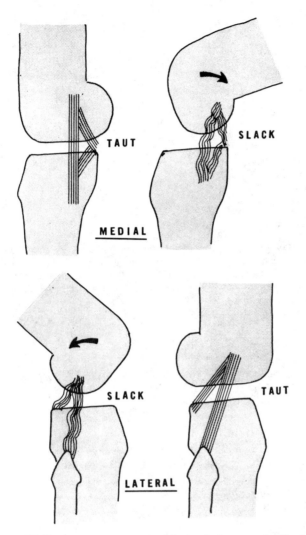

FIGURE 35. Ligamentous tautness and laxity during extension-flexion.

The ligaments aid in knee extension. When the tibia is fixed from the foot being weight bearing, the anterior cruciate acts as a guide wire as the knee approaches full extension. When the femur is fixed, the anterior cruciate controls lateral rotation of the tibia. As the knee moves from flexion to extension, the motion of the lateral condyle is stopped at 160° by the anterior cruciate and the lateral collateral ligament. Continued quadriceps contraction causes the medial condyle to move the additional 20° (to full 180°) and externally rotates the tibia upon the femur.

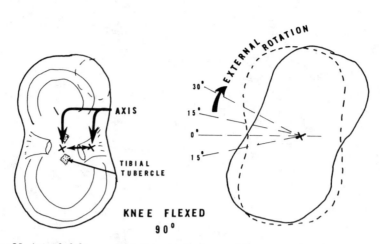

FIGURE 36. Axis of gliding and rotation. As the femur glides upon the tibia, the axis of axial rotation shifts. The degree of axial rotation varies according to the degree of flexion. None (0°) is possible at full extension or complete hyperflexion. Gradual rotation is possible until 90° of flexion is reached: 30 to 40° of rotation is possible at this point of flexion with more external rotation than internal.

BIBLIOGRAPHY

DEANDRADE, JR, GRANT, C, AND ST JOHN, D: *A joint distension and reflex muscle inhibition in the knee.* J Bone Joint Surg 47-A(2):313, 1965.

HELFET, AJ: *Function of the cruciate ligaments of the knee-joint.* Lancet May 1:665, 1948.

HONNOR, R AND THOMPSON, RC: *The nutritional pathways of articular cartilage.* J Bone Joint Surg 53-A(4):742, June 1971.

KENNEDY, JC, WEINBERG, HW, AND WILSON, AS: *The anatomy and function of the anterior cruciate ligament.* J Bone Joint Surg 56-A(2):223, March 1974.

LIEB, FJ AND PERRY, J: *Quadriceps function. An electromyographic study under isometric conditions.* J Bone Joint Surg 53-A(4):749, June 1971.

MARSHALL, JL, GIRGIS, FG, AND ZELKO, RR: *The biceps femoris tendon and its functional significance.* J Bone Joint Surg 54-A(7):1444, October 1972.

PARÉ, EB, STERN, JT, AND SCHWARTZ, JW: *Functional differentiation within the tensor fasciae latae.* J Bone Joint Surg 63-A(9):1457, December 1981.

WALKER, PS AND ERKMAN, MJ: *The role of the menisci in force transmission across the knee.* Clin Orthop 109:184, June 1975.

CHAPTER 3

Meniscus Injuries

Many factors are involved in injury of a meniscus. The exact pathomechanics is not always clearly ascertained by a careful history nor an exacting examination.

The medial meniscus sustains injury more often than does the lateral in a ratio of 3 to 1. Smillie places the injury in athletes as 3 to 1 but other authors place it as high as 8 to 1. Injury of the medial over the lateral meniscus in miners has been placed as high as 20 to 1. The difference in ratios is correlated to the particular movements and positions of these varied professions and activities.

In studying mechanical etiologic factors, it is considered that damage to the meniscus occurs from compressive or traction forces or a combination of both. Injury results from weight bearing upon the knee combined with faulty, forceful, or excessive motion either in flexion-rotation or extension-rotation. The combination of weight bearing *with* rotatory stress during flexion or extension as a cause of meniscus injury appears to be well accepted.

In previous chapters, it was stated that the fully extended knee with normal musculature and ligamentous structure is stable. No significant lateral nor rotatory motion is possible unless an overwhelming force tears the ligaments or causes a fracture or dislocation.

During normal motion, flexion is accompanied by internal rotation of the tibia upon the femur—extension accompanied by external rotation. The ligaments alternately slacken or become taut; the menisci move appropriately forward in extension and backward in flexion.

The medial meniscus, being firmly attached around its entire periphery, moves less than the lateral meniscus, which is more centrally attached. By virtue of greater mobility, the lateral meniscus sustains less injury.

During flexion and extension of the knee, the menisci move anteriorly and posteriorly respectively. With maximum flexion, the posterior portions of the menisci are compressed between the posterior aspects of the tibial and femoral condyles. Internal rotation of the femur upon the tibia in this flexed position will force the posterior segment of the medial meniscus toward the center of the joint space. Sudden extension of the knee can trap its posterior horn and create traction upon the entrapped meniscus. A longitudinal tear results in the meniscus (Fig. 37). The more mobile lateral meniscus can escape this entrapment and subsequent longitudinal tear.

External rotation of the femur upon the tibia in the bent knee position displaces the posterior horn of the lateral meniscus toward the center of the joint. Extension of the knee in this position of rotation, contrary to the resultant injury to the medial meniscus, does not cause a longitudinal tear but rather straightens (elongates) the lateral meniscus, placing strain upon the inner concave margin of the meniscus and tearing it transversely or obliquely (see Fig. 37).

Tearing of the meniscus with the knee fully extended is rare unless the tearing is a part of an extensive injury that disrupts the cruciate or collateral ligaments with or without condylar fracture.

The causative mechanism, therefore, must be considered to be flexion and extension of the knee, combined with forceful internal or external rotation that occurs when the tibia is fixed to the ground in a weight-bearing posture; thus the leg cannot avoid or minimize the torsion stress. From the crouched position with knees fully flexed or even hyperflexed, the femur must internally rotate upon the tibia during re-extension to the erect posture.

Another theory postulated to explain the mechanism of meniscus tear is that, combined with flexion and external rotation, a *forced valgus* of the knee (Fig. 38) occurs in which the medial joint space is opened. The opposing femoral and tibial condyle now grasp (as would a pair of pliers) the entrapped meniscus, which intrudes into the open medial joint space. The meniscus is crushed, creating a longitudinal tear and displacing the inner fragment of the posterior horn into the joint. This theory is made more plausible because the deeper, more concave surface of the medial tibial articular condyle allows easier access of the meniscus into this space (see Fig. 1).

A complete longitudinal tear is rare in an initial injury to a normal meniscus but may be extended by repeated injuries. This sequence is questioned by some authorities. The fact that the undersurface of the meniscus reveals the early site of damage is probably explained by the fact that the cartilage moves with the femur, thus causing irritation by the tibial surface.

Undoubtedly, there are other factors, such as constitutional inadequacy, ligamentous laxity, muscular inadequacy, faulty stressful work habits, obesity, excessive knee valgus or varus that place unequal stress upon knee

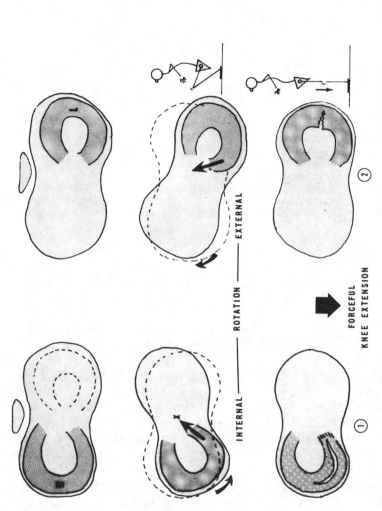

FIGURE 37. Mechanism of meniscus tear. *1*, With the knee fully flexed and the femur *internally* rotated, the medial meniscus is displaced posteriorly and the posterior horn (X) moves toward the center. Forceful extension of the knee causes a longitudinal tearing because of the meniscus capsular attachment or tear of the posterior attachment, or both. *2*, With the knee fully flexed and the femur *externally* rotated, the lateral meniscus is moved posteriorly and its posterior horn toward the center of the joint. Forceful knee extension *elongates* the meniscus, causing radial tearing on the medial (inner) margin of the meniscus.

43

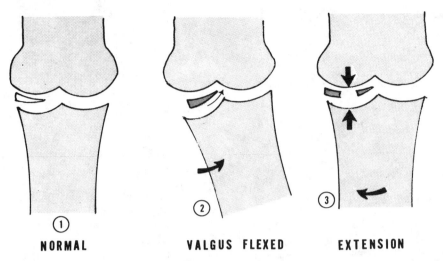

| NORMAL | VALGUS FLEXED | EXTENSION |

FIGURE 38. Valgus theory of meniscus tear. The combination of knee flexion with forced valgus, which opens the medial aspect of the knee joint, plus the deeper, more concave, tibial condyle, forces the meniscus toward the center of the joint. Re-extension pinches the entrapped meniscus between the opposing condyles.

structures, and violent sports, that contribute to meniscus tear and degenerative changes. Most of these ideas are conjectural but plausible. Frequently unrecognized meniscus injury occurs concurrently with tibial plateau fractures when the presence of the fracture obscures the meniscus lesion.

CLINICAL-PATHOLOGIC CONCEPTS

The initial tear of the medial meniscus occurs most often in the posterior pole. If the longitudinal tear occurs exclusively in the posterior third of the meniscus, by virtue of its inherent elasticity, the meniscus springs back into its normal position.

If the tear is extensive and extends anteriorly past the collateral ligament, it bunches up between the two condyles and causes a locking of the knee joint.

In an extensive tear, the entire inner fragment may be displaced to the center of the joint, in which case no locking results because the central fragment resides in the intercondylar fossa (Fig. 39).

Symptoms are *not* caused by the cartilage tear per se but by stretching or tearing its peripheral attachments and the acute synovial reaction within the joint space. The severity of the meniscus injury does *not* necessarily relate to the severity of the pain.

Synovial effusion invariably accompanies meniscus tears and results from injury to the synovium, capsule, or ligaments. It is not due to tear-

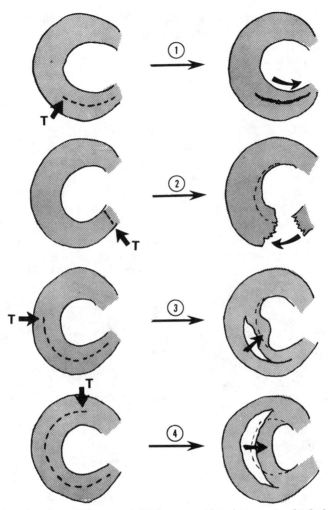

FIGURE 39. Types of meniscus tears. *1,* With a tear within the posterior third of the meniscus, the elasticity of the cartilage springs the meniscus back into its normal position. *2,* Posterior tear *(T)* of the horn's attachment causes the anterior portion to bunch, and locking results. *3,* A tear *(T)* halfway to the collateral ligament causes a bunching of the middle portion of the meniscus with similar symptoms to 2. *4,* If the tear *(T)* is complete (entire length of the meniscus), the central portion of the meniscus moves toward the center of the joint. This is called a bucket handle tear. No locking occurs because the central fragment is in the intercondylar fossa.

ing of the fibrocartilaginous meniscus. It must be remembered that knee injuries other than meniscus tears can cause effusion and must be considered in the differential diagnosis of a swollen knee. A large effusion may give the feeling of tightness with no pain. Hemarthrosis almost always gives severe pain.

Tears in the substance of the avascular portion of the cartilage *do not* heal. Tears in the peripheral zones heal by invasion of fibrous tissue. The meniscus removed by meniscectomy is replaced by dense collagen tissue from the remaining portion of the meniscus.

DIAGNOSTIC SIGNS AND SYMPTOMS

The history given by the patient or by an observer at the time of injury is often that of a twisting, turning movement of the leg with the foot firmly fixed to the ground (as in an athlete's quick turn in a running event), a direct blow to the turned flexed extremity, or coming to an erect posture from a full crouched position. The exact history may not be evident to the patient who attributes the injury to the fall that follows the meniscus knee injury.

Pain is usually severe and sudden as if "something tore within the knee." Pain from an acute tear of the meniscus usually causes immediate cessation of activity, whereas a ligamentous sprain permits continuation albeit with discomfort. Swelling occurs within hours and occasionally the knee locks immediately but the locking may be momentary and suddenly, spontaneously, reduced.

Effusion is usually present following the initial injury. Without effusion, an extra-articular lesion must be suspected. Lesions of the lateral meniscus cause less effusion than the medial cartilage because of having less peripheral capsular attachment. Immediate massive bloody effusion implies severe capsular, ligamentous or bony injury, or a combination of both.

Tenderness may be elicited along the entire joint line, which probably indicates tearing of the peripheral attachment of the meniscus. Tenderness is present mostly in the posterior area of the knee joint. Rarely is there tenderness anteriorly as tearing usually does not occur there. In meniscus tear, tenderness may be in the region of the medial collateral ligament but tear of the ligament, with or without associated meniscus injury, causes tenderness *above* the joint line.

Locking is rare in an initial injury as the tear is usually in the posterior third of the meniscus with no displacement or bunching of the cartilage (see Fig. 39). In more severe initial tears or repeated tearing injuries, which extend anteriorly to or past the coronal plane of the joint, locking can result, thus preventing *full extension of the knee.* True locking is usually sudden and unlocking may be equally sudden. Gradual locking may be the result of effusion hemorrhage within the infrapatellar fat pad or from an unrecognized loose body within the joint. Not all meniscus injuries give a history of locking; in fact, 50 percent of these injuries have never locked.

Buckling, giving away of the knee, noted by the patient during walking, often on irregular terrain, may indicate a tear of the posterior segment of the meniscus.

Clicking, audible to the patient or examiner, is considered to be caused by the femoral condyle riding over an articular irregularity. It must be differentiated from the grating noted in an osteoarthritic knee, in chondromalacia patellae, or when the hamstring tendon snaps over the femoral condyle.

Quadriceps Atrophy

Atrophy of the quadriceps occurs rapidly after a meniscus injury and is noted particularly in the vastus medialis. It has been claimed that in the absence of atrophy a meniscus injury or an internal knee derangement has probably not occurred. Atrophy is measurably verified within days after an injury and is noted within 10 to 14 days. Measurement of the thigh is a mandatory aspect of every knee injury and examination (Fig. 40).

Effusion of the knee joint leads to *reflex inhibition* of the quadriceps through a neurologic mechanism not well understood. It is either the pain or the distension of the capsule that produces the inibition of quadriceps contraction. All joints of the body, hence also the knee, will assume the position of minimal joint (intra-articular) pressure. In the knee, midflexion has the minimum of pressure that increases by extension. The patient apparently assumes a midflexed position and avoids extension to avoid increased intra-articular pressure (Fig. 41). The increased pressure on the capsule, which is well supplied by pain and pressure fibers, can well stimulate reflex innervation.

Clinical Meniscus Signs

So-called *meniscus signs* are numerous and vary depending upon the author being studied. Unfortunately, these signs employ the proper name of the physician who initially described that particular test. A physiologic basis for any test makes the examination and its interpretation more meaningful.

MCMURRAY SIGN. This is a time-honored test in which the patient in the recumbent position has the knee flexed until the heel touches (or approaches) the buttocks (Fig. 42). To test the medial meniscus, the leg is externally rotated upon the femur (internally rotated to test the lateral meniscus). The leg is gradually extended with rotation forcefully maintained. The test is valid only during extension from 90° of flexion and does not diagnose tears in the anterior one third of the meniscus.

47

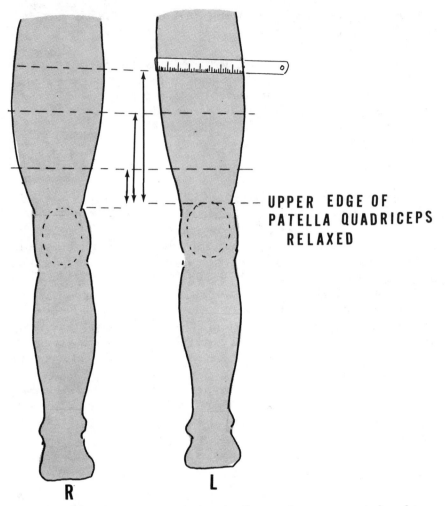

UPPER EDGE OF
PATELLA QUADRICEPS
RELAXED

R   L

FIGURE 40. Quadriceps measurement for atrophy. Comparative measurement of quadriceps circumference is done at measured distances (4, 6, 8, 10, and 12 inches) from upper edge of patella with quadriceps relaxed.

APLEY TEST. This test aims at differentiating a meniscus lesion from capsular or ligamentous injury. With the patient prone, the knee is flexed to 90° and the leg is rotated with simultaneous upward traction. Pain with this maneuver implies capsular or ligamentous injury. Rotation of the bent knee with downward pressure causing pain or "clicking" indicates a meniscus lesion (see Fig. 42).

STEINMANN'S TENDERNESS DISPLACEMENT SIGN. Tenderness is displaced posteriorly as the knee is flexed, anteriorly as the knee is extended (Fig.

48

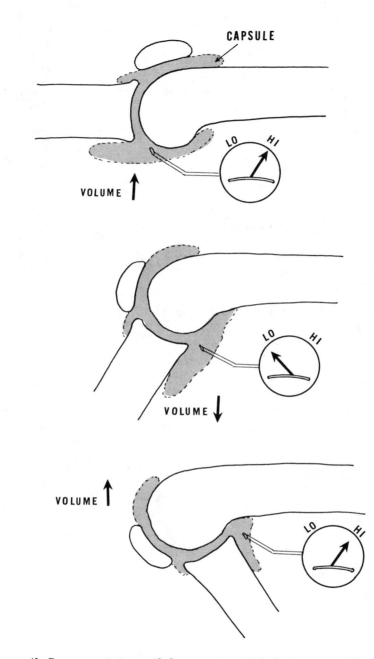

FIGURE 41. Pressure variations with knee position. With the knee in midflexed position *(middle)*, there is the lowest pressure, thus less irritation of sensory (pain) and pressure nerves. This is the position assumed by the patient who avoids full extension *(top)* or further flexion *(bottom)*.

49

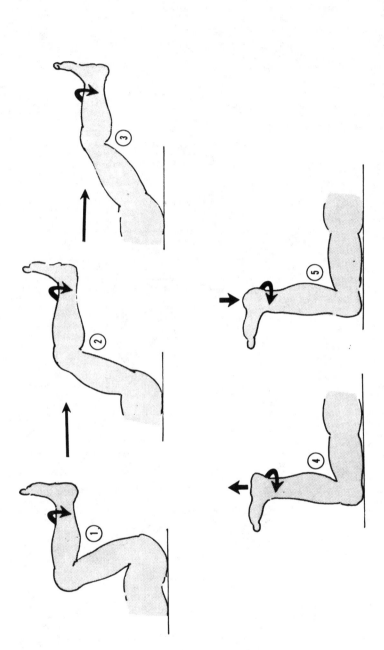

FIGURE 42. Meniscus signs (examination). *1, 2, 3, McMurray test.* The patient is supine with knee fully flexed, heel touching the buttocks at the start. The leg is internally rotated for lateral meniscus testing or externally rotated for medial meniscus testing. Then the knee is fully extended. A painful click occurs if there is a meniscus lesion. The test is more meaningful in the first phase of knee extension. Full extension limitation does not indicate an anterior meniscus lesion. *4, 5, Apley test.* The patient is prone. Leg is internally or externally rotated with simultaneous traction. Pain indicates a capsular or ligamentous lesion. Rotation with downward pressure that causes pain indicates meniscus lesion.

50

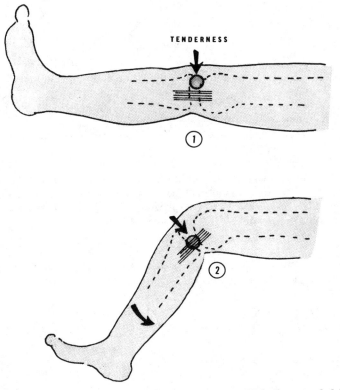

FIGURE 43. Meniscus sign: tenderness displacement test. *1*, With the extended knee, the tenderness over the medial meniscus occurs anteriorly. *2*, As the knee is flexed the tenderness migrates posteriorly toward the medial collateral ligament.

43). The site of tenderness does not shift in degenerative osteoarthrosis of the knee.

HYPERFLEXION MENISCUS TEST. With the patient prone, hyperflexing the knee (Fig. 44) with the lower leg in internal or external rotation may cause the cartilage to slip forward and cause a painful click as the opposing condyles compress the fragment.

There are many other tests for meniscus lesions but all are founded on the same mechanical basis. With the understanding of the mechanics of the underlying pathology, examiners should familiarize themselves with proper consistent examination and become proficient in a careful technique in order to assure a meaningful examination.

Arthrography

The diagnostic procedure of injecting dye into the joint and thus outlining all intra-articular tissues is gaining more advocates and is becoming a

51

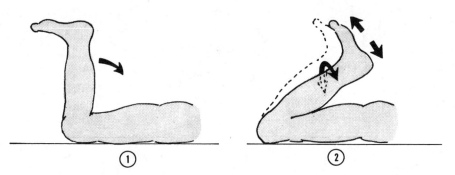

FIGURE 44. Hyperflexion meniscus test. With the patient prone, the knee is flexed to 90°. Then, with internal or external rotation of the leg upon the femur, the knee is *hyperflexed*. Painful clicking may indicate a posterior meniscus tear. Doing this maneuver may cause the knee to lock from movement of the fragment into the joint.

gratifying procedure. Full detail and discussion of the numerous interpretations made possible by this test is beyond the scope of this book but certain principals are indicated.

Many pitfalls that may lead to faulty diagnosis or unwarranted negative conclusions exist in the interpretation of an arthrogram. Therefore, the test should be performed and interpreted by an experienced diagnostic radiologist or trained orthopedist.

Before arthrography is performed, the joint should be evacuated as completely as possible of all intra-articular fluid. Air then is injected into the joint to distend the capsule and create a fluoroscopic contrast. Twenty to forty milliliters of air can safely and painlessly be injected, but the exact amount should be restricted to that amount that causes no painful distension yet good visible contrast in the joint. After the air is injected, 3 to 4 ml of liquid contrast medium is injected through the same needle. The needle is then withdrawn.

The patient is instructed to fully move the knee after the injection and should *not* put weight on that leg. However, the patient may stand on the other leg and allow the injected knee to be dependent. These numerous movements insure the dyecoating of all intra-articular tissues. Not only the menisci and intra-articular ligaments may be visualized but also the bursae that connect with the joint space. Several examples are graphically illustrated to explain the principals of arthrography (Figs. 45 and 46). Currently, much literature on the subject is being published.

TREATMENT

Tears into the meniscus that do not extend into the peripheral vascular portion of the fibrocartilage do not heal. Those that do extend into the

52

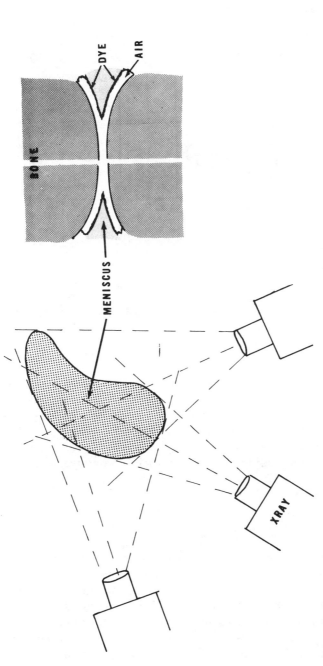

FIGURE 45. Arthrography: The knee, and thus the meniscus, is rotated before the x-ray so that both poles and the entire meniscus are visualized. *Left*, The lateral and medial aspects of the joint are visualized separately; *Right*, The air creates contrast and the dye coats all intra-articular tissues.

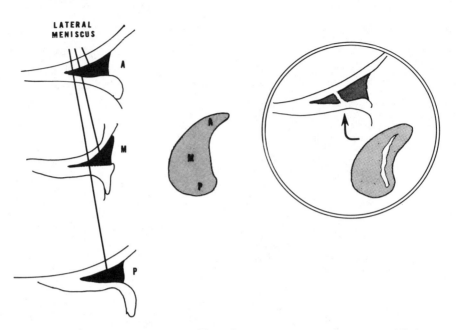

FIGURE 46. Arthrograms. *Center,* Normal lateral menisci: *A,* Anterior horn; *M,* Middle horn; *P,* Posterior horn. *Left,* What is seen on lateral x-ray films; *Right,* An arthrogram taken of a torn meniscus.

vascular zone heal if there is reduction of the displaced meniscus and the knee is immobilized for at least three weeks. In an obvious tear, that is, one with incomplete extension indicating medial displacement, conservative treatment must be viewed as temporary, permitting merely painfree return of function, but futile if disability and pain recur.

The decision regarding surgery varies with the surgeon's experience and no hard-fast rules are applicable. In general, however, the locking knee with recurrences should have arthrotomy.

Reduction

The locked knee must be reduced within 24 hours. After this time, the effusion causes a loss of elasticity of the meniscus and prevents its springing back into normal position. This reduction manipulation (Fig. 47) usually does not require an anesthetic. The technique is (1) apply longitudinal traction with simultaneous rotation in both directions and lateral motion (valgus and varus stress) with leg principally in *valgus* position; (2) full flexion of the knee with forceful internal rotation if the medial meniscus is being treated, (external rotation if the lateral meniscus); and (3) forceful kicking (extension) by the patient. Achieving full free range of

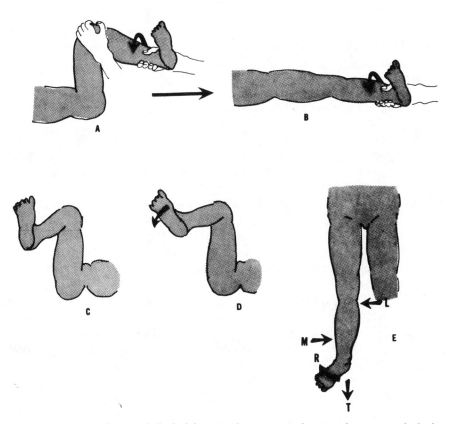

FIGURE 47. Manipulation of "locked knee." The purpose of manipulation to unlock the meniscus is to relieve pain and prevent further damage to the meniscus. A, In lateral meniscus, the knee is fully flexed and some pressure is exerted to cause varus of the leg (M, medial pressure; L, lateral pressure). D, The leg is externally rotated. Then the surgeon suddenly (but not forcefully) extends the leg A to B. For lesions of the medial meniscus the opposite motion (internal rotation varus) is used.

motion indicates a reduction (unlocking). The range must be compared with the other leg to ascertain full extension as compared to normal.

Repeated unsuccessful manipulations may cause extension of the tear anteriorly or centrally into the joint space (see Fig. 39). If there is persistence of a displaced fragment, the last few degrees of extension are both actively and passively prevented. *Forceful attempts must be avoided* and weight bearing should not be permitted.

Conservative Treatment

Conservative treatment is permissible; in fact, it is indicated if full extension is possible when a definite diagnosis is not possible immediately following the initial injury. A more careful examination is possible after the effusion has subsided, the quadriceps tone has returned, and function appears possible. If full range of motion is possible, ambulation for testing is permitted.

If manipulation has reduced the locking, a rehabilitation program of exercises (to be described later) may be started. Deep knee bends and squats are to be avoided as are sports activities.

In addition to a meniscus tear, there may be tearing or severe sprain of the collateral or cruciate ligamentous structures. An evaluation of these structures must be carefully made as well as performing the meniscus signs.

In the absence of locking, two or three weeks of conservative treatment will reduce or remove the effusion and permit accurate evaluation. If there is an associated ligamentous lesion *with* a locked knee, the knee must first be unlocked. The purpose of conservative treatment is to promote absorption of the effusion, restoration of the quadriceps mechanism, and immediate unlocking of the joint.

The unlocking has been described. Removal of the effusion is undertaken by initial application of ice packs for 24 to 36 hours, followed by heat (e.g., whirlpool, hot moist packs, diathermy), aspiration with or without simultaneous instillation of hyaluronidase, avoidance of weight bearing (through the use of crutches, wheel chair, and so forth), and avoidance of compression dressings. Quadriceps function maintenance or restoration is discussed in the postoperative section.

Surgery

Surgical technique is beyond the scope of this text and reference is made to the many excellent orthopedic texts and to scientific articles in orthopedic journals. Surgical failures in which the results are poor (e.g., knee instability, persistent pain and limitation, recurrent effusion) are caused by:

1. Improper or incomplete diagnosis.
2. Incompetent surgical technique.
3. Excessively prolonged conservative treatment with repeated episodes of locking or giving way.
4. Meniscus injury in a knee exhibiting severe degenerative osteoarthritic changes.
5. Removal of only *one* of the affected menisci.
6. Incomplete removal of the meniscus. (This indication is disputed in current literature.)
7. Inadequate postoperative treatment.

POSTOPERATIVE REHABILITATION PROGRAM. Immediately postoperative, before the tourniquet is removed, the leg should be firmly wrapped in a compression dressing and elevated. On the second day, quadriceps setting exercises should be started. These should be done for 10 to 15 minutes 3 to 4 times daily. When possible, at elective surgery or time permitting, instruction in these exercises *preoperatively* facilitates their being understood and properly done postoperatively. From the third day, the patient should progress from isometric exercises to straight leg raising, using the weight of the leg for resistance. Then should progress to increased resistance as tolerated with the encouragement and supervision so that failure to progress is not permitted. Excessive pain or effusion or a combination of both should cause review of the program. Normal use is usual within 10 weeks.

Quadriceps Exercises

Exercise to strengthen the quadriceps mechanism is of sufficient importance to devote space to a full discussion and detail. The question is that of power versus endurance: which to stress? How is it attainable? Which is important?

Power building exercises do not develop endurance, but power is essential and should be developed first. The rate of development of muscle volume (mass), and thus power, is proportional to the resistance imposed upon the muscle. Heavy resistance exercise with low repetition creates power; low resistance with high repetition creates endurance. The greater the stretch (elongation) of the muscle, the greater the contractile power; thus in the stretched position fewer fibers are used than when contraction is in the shortened position. Maximum tension occurs at lengths 10 percent longer than the resting length.

Strength increase occurs by the recruitment of additional motor units rather than by more rapid firing of the contracting units. Therefore, strength increase depends upon (1) greater voluntary effort, (2) integrity of the central nervous system, and (3) better synaptic and endplate functions. Only the first is directly influenced by patient effort.

Progressive resistive exercises are essentially rhythmic *dynamic* exercises. They use maximum resistance (load) and are gradually upgraded as strength improves. A prescribed increase in daily series moves the muscle through its full range of motion and insures proper positioning so that only the prime movers of that joint are treated.

Static (muscle setting) exercises have their greatest value where joint motion needs to be avoided or is not possible. *Isokinetic exercises* attempt a combination of isotonic (kinetic) and isometric (static) exercises in which speed of motion is kept constant by equipment and maximum tension is applied and maintained through the entire cycle.

The types of exercises and their exact application vary with the stage of the recovery or postoperative state. Early in postsprain condition, postoperatively when joint motion is not desired, or with leg in a pressure dressing or cast when joint motion is not wanted, *isometric setting exercises* are advisable. The term "isometric" is a misnomer, implying no movement when there is motion of the muscle and the patella. Only joint motion is excluded.

In chondromalacia patellae, where quadriceps exercises must be performed with minimal or no patellar movement, the quadriceps should be slowly and fully contracted before maximum contraction (setting) is attempted. Straight leg raising against resistance is effective here. With the leg fully extended, have the patient contract the quadriceps muscle to its maximum with the greatest effort tolerated. Motion is judged by observing the upward motion of the patella, bulging or firming of the quadriceps muscle. The contraction should be sustained for a count to three or five, then relaxed. This exercise is performed 15 to 30 times every hour of the waking day with attempt at increasing the effort of contraction.

Straight leg raising without resistance is begun when setting has been mastered and strength, as observed by muscle bulk, appears to be returning. Straight leg raising should be done hourly with sustained elevation at 45° and an intermittent rest period. Studies (Ladley) show that this straight leg raising is a less effective progressive form of exercise than resisted extension with knee slightly flexed over a supporting block (Fig. 48).

Straight leg raising against elastic resistance or sand bags of graded weights are then instituted. Postoperative resistance exercises are not started for three to four weeks after surgery but setting exercises should be started the first postoperative day, with straight leg raising begun as soon as tolerated by the patient even though the leg may be in a pressure dressing or cast.

Progress to resistance exercises of a kinetic type (with range of motion of the joint) is based on certain concepts and approved methods. Resistance is applied either manually by a physical therapist or trained relative or with mechanical equipment. Several concepts need clarification before the progressive resistive program is detailed. As stated previously, quadriceps setting with knee fully extended is not considered to be the most effective method. By placing a small, well-padded block of less than 3 inches in thickness under the knee and flexing the knee very slightly, exercise seems more effective as ascertained by electromyographic surface electrodes (see Fig. 48). The position or action of the foot, simultaneous plantar flexion, dorsiflexion, inversion, or eversion during quadriceps ex-

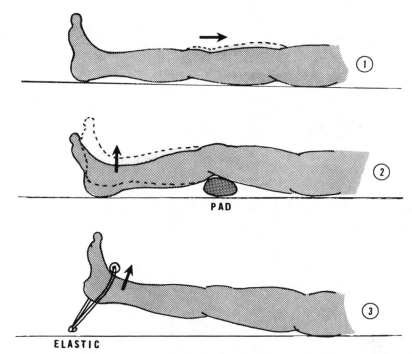

FIGURE 48. Types of quadriceps exercises. *1,* Setting or isometric exercises with knee fully extended. Joint does not move but muscle shortens: patella moves up. *2,* Isometric (kinetic) exercise. With a 3-inch thick pad under the knee the quadriceps contracts. The joint range of motion is minimal and quadriceps function is enhanced over *1.* *3,* Increase in exercise with an elastic strap to resist straight leg raising.

ercises have been questioned. It appears that concurrent ankle dorsiflexion enhances the quadriceps efficiency.

The essence of progressive resistance exercise (PRE) (Delorme) is the determination of the maximum resistance that the patient can overcome to full extension for one contraction (called 1 RM) and the determination of the weight that can be lifted to full extension for 10 repeated efforts (10 RM). As the program progresses, the weight of 10 RM attached to the foot and allowed to rest on a support between lifts is raised to full knee extension and then lowered slowly back to the support for a period of rest for one to two minutes. It is again lifted. At the extreme of full extension, maximum effort is exerted to recruit all motor units and the leg is held extended for the count of three. The exercise period lasts 30 to 45 minutes and is done 3 times a day. Heat and massage is beneficial following each series.

The resistance is gradually increased and the repetitions decreased. The 10 RMs are determined every week, with increase in increments of ¼ to

59

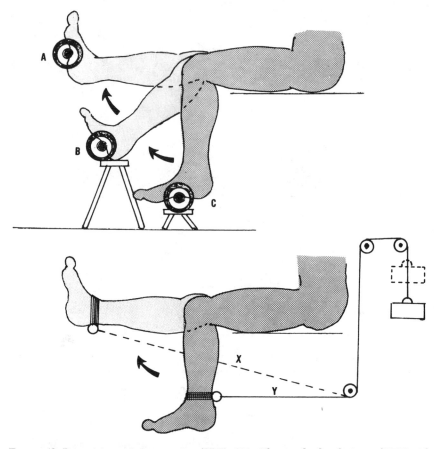

FIGURE 49. Progressive resistive exercises (PRE). *Top*, The standard technique of PRE with a weighted boot. Full extension is attempted *(A)* and briefly sustained. *B*, The leg is lowered until the weight and foot are supported to prevent ligamentous stress. *B* causes exercise toward extension from the semi-extended position, where the vastus medialis is most effective, rather than from *C*, where resistance against the quadriceps is minimal as the weight pulls vertically along the tibial shaft. In the *C* position there is a greater chance of stress upon the ligaments of the knee from the weighted dependent leg. *Bottom*, Resistance with pulleys and weights places maximum resistance in the first 45° of extension *(Y)* and decreases as the leg extends, thus placing none (0°) at full extension *(X)*.

$1/2$ lb as tolerated up to 1 lb. Gradually, a weight that permits merely one full excursion is reached; this is 1 RM and requires maximum effort. This lift is done three times daily and followed by rest, heat, and massage if desired. This weight is also gradually increased. A weight of 30 to 35 lb can be reached in most adults; more in athletes. Normal power is usually reached in three to six weeks.

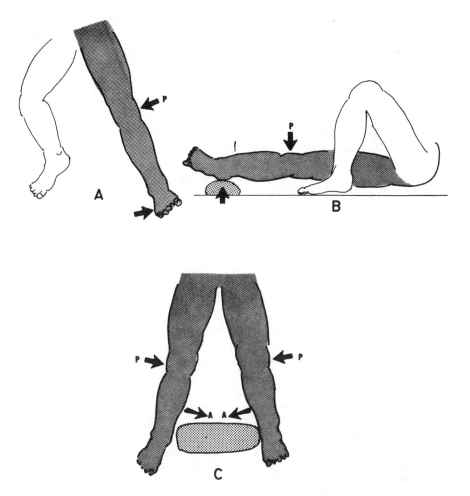

FIGURE 50. Exercises to stress ligaments of the knee. Both medial and lateral collateral ligaments are stretched daily as part of the exercise program on the assumption that gentle but firm and repeated stress upon the ligaments increases their resilience. *A and B* indicate how the patient stretches manually the medial ligament. *C*, With the use of a firm pillow both active *(A)* and passive *(P)* exercises stretch and stress the ligaments. Exercises weighted against gravity also stress and strengthen ligaments.

Power having been or being reached, it is now desirable that endurance exercises be initiated. These include bicycling, stair climbing and descending, jumping jacks, shallow knee bends *(never to exceed 50 percent of a full squat)*, and jogging.

The use of a weight applied to the foot-ankle rather than the use of a pulley needs clarification (Fig. 49). Resistance from the weighted boot is

61

maximum in the most effective range of extension, the last 45°. By lowering the boot to the support after each lift, no ligamentous strain or stretch to the ligaments occurs. The resistance from the pulley is maximum at the beginning of knee extension when the knee is flexed 90° but decreases as the knee extends.

Exercises are also considered to be effective in increasing the tensile strength of ligaments. As the quadriceps' power returns, gentle stress upon the ligaments should be incorporated in the exercise program (Fig. 50). *Gentle* manual pressure upon the leg in a valgus or varus direction is taught the patient, in addition to side-lying, abduction-adduction exercises against a weighted boot. Prone progressive resistance exercises to the hamstrings are beneficial.

BIBLIOGRAPHY

COOPER, RA: *Knee arthrography meniscal and extrameniscal lesions.* Orthopedics 4(10):1150, October 1981.

DELORME, TL: *Restoration of muscle power by heavy resistance exercises.* J Bone Joint Surg 27:645, 1945.

DICKINSON, AL: *Resistance exercises for development of strength of muscles that extend leg at knee: A comparative study of three methods.* PhD Dissertation. State University of Iowa, Iowa City, 1962.

ERAT, K AND NOBLE, J: *In defense of the meniscus.* J Bone Joint Surg 62-B(1):7, February 1980.

EYRING, EJ AND MURRAY, WR: *The effect of joint position on the pressure of intra-articular effusion.* J Bone Joint Surg 46-A(6):1235, September 1964.

IRELAND, J, TRICKEY, EL, AND STOKER, DJ: *Arthroscopy and arthrography of the knee. A critical review.* J Bone Joint Surg 62-B(1):3, February 1980.

KING, D: *The healing of semilunar cartilage.* J Bone Joint Surg 18:333, 1936.

KLEIN, KK: *A continuation study of specific progressive resistance exercises for increasing medial lateral collateral ligamentous stability.* J Assoc Physical Mental Rehab 19:162, 1965.

LADLEY, G: *An investigation into the effectiveness of various forms of quadriceps exercises.* Physiotherapy 57:356, 1971.

SCHAER, H: *Der Meniscusschaden.* G Thieme, Leipsig, 1938.

WEINGARDEN, ST, LOUIS, LD, AND WAYLONIS, GW: *Electromyographic changes in postmeniscectomy patients.* JAMA 241(12):1248, March 22, 1979.

WEISEL, A: *Don't throw away the meniscus.* Orthopaedic Review Vol X(11):121, November 1981.

CHAPTER 4

Ligamentous-Capsular Injuries

Ligaments are fibrous collagen tissues properly employed about a joint to prevent abnormal or excessive motion of that joint. Excessive joint motion that causes injury to the ligaments constitutes a *sprain*. Sprains may vary from complete tear of the ligament, with or without avulsion of the fragment of bone to which it is attached, to merely minor tearing of a few fibers without loss of integrity of the ligament. Tears within a ligament may be longitudinal, transverse, or oblique, causing elongation of the remaining ligamentous fibers. *Strain* semantically may be considered to be the physical force imposed upon the ligamentous tissues possibly exceeding normal stress but not causing deformation or damage to the tissues. Physiologic recovery is expected.

The knee joint sustains a sprain when a force (strain) is exerted that exceeds normal range of motion or causes an abnormal motion of the joint with tissue injury. Abnormal motion includes abduction or adduction of the extended knee, excessive rotation, hyperextension or hyperflexion, or any combination of the above. The patient may be able to describe the exact type and severity of the injury sustained and a witness may furnish the necessary details. Frequently, neither the patient nor the witness can furnish a significant history because its significance at the time of insult is not so considered by the patient until specifically questioned.

Immediate evaluation of the injured knee is desirable because specific treatment is dependent on the severity of the injury. Was the injury considered serious by the patient? Was the patient totally disabled immediately or could the activity be continued? Was the pain mild or severe? Did the knee lock? Was effusion immediate and marked or delayed and gradual? These details indicate the severity of ligamentous injury, meniscus involvement, and so forth. Later, after initial injury, secondary factors of pain, effusion, guarding, concern, and faulty memory all become confusing and render the history inaccurate.

CLASSIFICATION OF DEGREE OF STRAIN

Determination of the *degree* of ligamentous injury is necessary in order to initiate proper early treatment and give a reasonable prognosis as to ultimate functional recovery, need for surgery, or ultimate duration of rehabilitation, or a combination of these. Ligamentous injuries are generally classified as mild, moderate, or severe. The following classification obviously is arbitrary with much overlap and dependent upon the experience of the examiner. Basically it is:

Mild: A few fibers are torn but the integrity of the ligament is maintained and the joint remains stable.
Moderate: Fibers are torn in sufficient quantity to diminish the ligamentous function but still maintain joint stability. Some excessive joint motion is evident when compared to the other side, with some discomfort elicited.
Severe: Complete tearing of fibers with loss of integrity and evidence of joint instability.

Diagnostic Features and Treatment

Injury to the ligamentous structure is commonplace, painful, and potentially disabling. Thorough knowledge of the functional anatomy and the tests needed to evaluate the integrity of the ligaments justifies some repetition. The medial and lateral collateral and cruciate ligaments have been discussed in Chapter 1. The functional anatomy of the ligament was discussed in Chapter 2. Further discussion here will attempt to relate injury to ligaments and their examination.

CRUCIATE LIGAMENTS

The cruciate ligaments are valuable stabilizers of the knee, which not only assist in knee flexion and extension but limit rotation as well as extension-flexion. Their function merits deeper study. The anterior cruciate ligament varies in length from 3.7 to 4.1 cm with an average of 3.9 cm. This ligament is taut when the knee is in full extension and when the knee is fully externally rotated at the femorotibial joint. It remains taut until 5 to 20° flexion and then relaxes. It is most relaxed at 40 to 50° flexion and becomes taut when the knee flexes to 70 to 90° (Fig. 51).

Rotation (internal) increases the tension of the anterior cruciate ligament even when the knee is flexed to 40 to 50°; the point at which the anterior cruciate ligament is most relaxed. External rotation increases the tautness of the ligament as does abduction of the knee. Anterior shear of the tibia upon the femur is permitted to 5 mm distance but then is

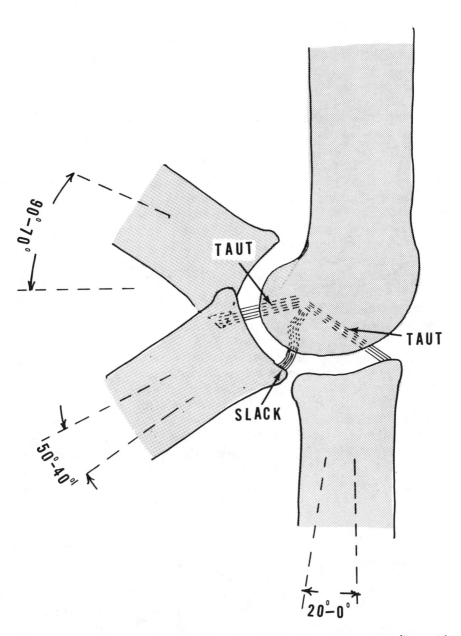

90°-70°

TAUT

TAUT

SLACK

50°-40°

20°-0°

FIGURE 51. Anterior cruciate ligament during knee flexion. The anterior cruciate ligament is taut at full (0°) extension and remains so until 20° flexion. It becomes maximally slack at 40 to 50° flexion, then again becomes taut at 70 to 80° flexion.

checked. Excessive external rotation can tear the anterior cruciate ligament, especially if there is added abduction. Hyperextension and anterior shear also may tear this ligament. With the knee flexed to 90° and externally rotated to 40 to 50°, the first limiting soft tissue that tears is the deep medial capsular ligament. Further rotation and abduction, the next tissue to tear is the tibial medial collateral ligament, then the anterior cruciate ligament (Fig. 52). Isolated tears of the anterior cruciate ligament, when they do happen, probably occur from a posterior force causing shear stress but also may occur from internal rotation.

In athletic injuries, the anterior cruciate ligament can be torn as an isolated injury, an acute deceleration from a sharp "stop and cut" movement. As the forward movement of the person is abruptly halted, the quadriceps decelerates the leg and simultaneously pulls the tibia forward upon the femur. This shear disrupts the anterior cruciate ligament (Fig. 53). Along with abrupt stop, the athlete frequently makes a rapid rotation ("cut") to form the direction of movement. This places anterior shear *and* rotatory stress upon the knee. The rotational stress depends upon which direction the "cut" is. After a jump, the knee absorbs the impact being slightly flexed, thus shear occurs at this point also due to deceleration. Typically, the athlete who is making the cut or lands after a jump feels a "pop" and the knee "giving way" and swelling occurs within three or four hours.

To prevent the injury, the athlete must be trained to increase the turn arc, that is, make more rounded turns. Quadricep exercises to increase the strength of the quadriceps *will not* protect the athletes cruciate ligament. Drills to teach rounded turn techniques are more efficient and teach the athlete to "stop" in two to three small steps rather than one step, which places stress of the tibia upon the femur (Fig. 54).

The anterior cruciate ligament tears mostly in its midportion, rarely at its long attachment. The blood supply of the cruciate ligament is from the middle geniculate artery and is sparce. The shape of the collagen fascicles and the tortuous blood vessels explain the slight elasticity of this ligament (Fig. 55).

In examining an injured knee in which a cruciate ligament is torn, the meniscus must also be suspected to be torn. In excessive rotatory instability noted during examination of the injured knee, the initial injury occurs in the medial capsular ligament, especially if the injury is that of severe abduction with the knee flexed. With the knee flexed, the vertical fibers of the tibial medial collateral ligaments have migrated posterior to axis of rotation and is slack causing the deep capsular ligament to receive the major impact of the valgus strain. As the medial capsular ligament tears, the pivotal point of rotation shifts laterally allowing the tibia to move anteriorly and laterally. As this tibial migration occurs, the anterior cruci-

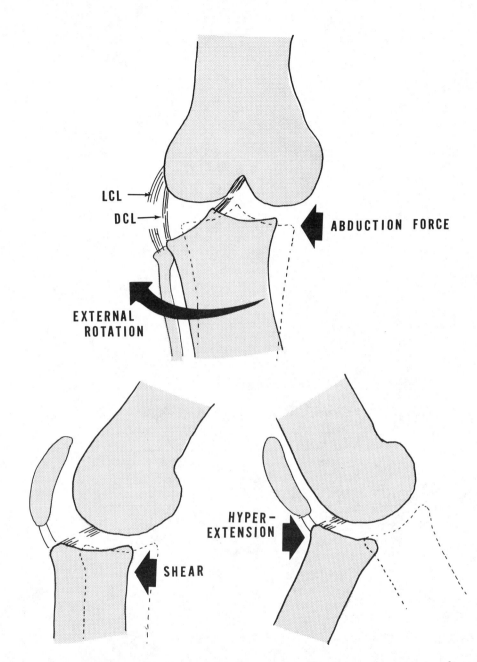

FIGURE 52. Mechanisms of anterior cruciate ligament tear. *Top,* Injury of severe external rotation with abduction injury. The lateral collateral ligament *(LCL)* tears first, then the deep capsular ligament *(DCL),* last is the tear of the anterior cruciate ligament. Anterior shear and severe hypertension of the knee can also tear the anterior cruciate ligament.

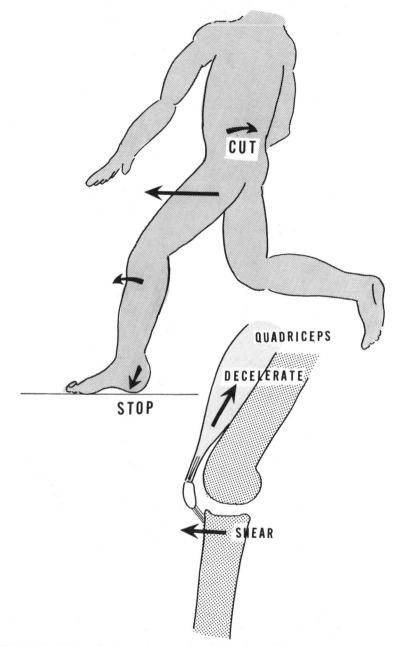

FIGURE 53. "Stop and cut" mechanism of athletic injury. Coming to an abrupt stop, with or without simultaneous rotation ("cut") places shear stress on the knee. The quadriceps abruptly decelerates the knee flexion placing added shear stress on the knee. Added "cut" adds rotatory stress upon the knee. Quadriceps deceleration causes anterior cruciate ligament shear. Deceleration is the "culprit".

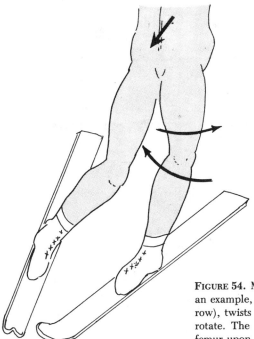

FIGURE 54. Mechanism of rotatory knee injury. As an example, a skier on downward glide (thick arrow), twists body to the left. The left ski does not rotate. The leg at the knee externally rotates the femur upon the tibia.

ate tenses, gets forced around the lateral femoral condyle and finally ruptures (see Fig. 31).

Clinical Testing

1. Varus-valgus (medial-lateral) stability is checked with the knee extended then flexed 20°, this tests the collateral ligaments.
2. With knee flexed and foot fixed, anterior posterior shear tests the cruciates.
3. The knee rotation is then checked for rotatory stability. With the knee flexed to 90° and the foot plantigrade on the table, the lower leg is internally rotated, then externally rotated—the degree measured and the left leg compared to the right. There should be no dependency of the leg placing gravity effect upon the ligaments.
4. With the tibia internally rotated, the lateral ligaments tense enough to prevent anterior-posterior (shear) movement *even* with complete tear of the medial ligaments and tear of the anterior cruciate ligament.
5. With 15° external rotation of the tibia, there is relaxation of the medial ligaments and the cruciate ligament. This 15° rotation is the beginning point of rotatory instability test.

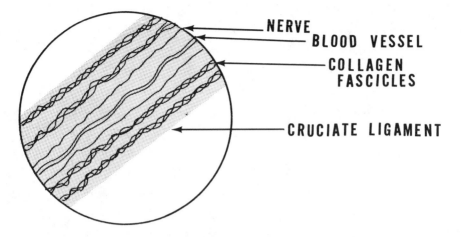

FIGURE 55. Microscopic view of cruciate ligament. The collagenous fascicles are undulated in a slight manner allowing little elongation. The blood vessels are tortuous but again slight. There are nerves within the ligament that subserve pain sensation. The structure explains the limited elasticity of the cruciate ligament.

6. Anterior posterior shear is then tested and rated as follows:

Normal laxity	0
Anterior dislocation of ½ inch	+1
Anterior dislocation of ½ to ¾ inch	+2
Anterior dislocation of ¾ inch or more	+3

As shown in Figure 56 the patient is recumbent with knee flexed to 90°. Examiner sits on the plantigrade foot. The tibia is rotated 15° internally, then 15° externally, then the tibia is pulled forward upon the femur. With the tibia externally rotated, the anterior cruciate ligament is relaxed as are the lateral ligaments, thus excessive anterior displacement of the tibia (a "positive" test) indicates medial capsular ligament disruption. The opposite leg must be similarly examined for comparison, assuming the opposite leg is normal.

MILD SPRAIN. Pain can be elicited by stress upon the ligaments. There is tenderness, and some local swelling is noted. The joint is stable with no effusion or locking. Certain movements that place stress on the joint may be painful.

Treatment is essentially the relief of discomfort by restricting activities and applying ice packs initially, followed by heat, compression wrapping, and oral medication of any anti-inflammatory agent. Local injection of an anesthetic agent with or without steroids may be desirable. Oral analgesics and injection can camouflage a more severe injury and permit aggravation. Activity may be permitted if the activity is not too stressful and the patient is reliable.

70

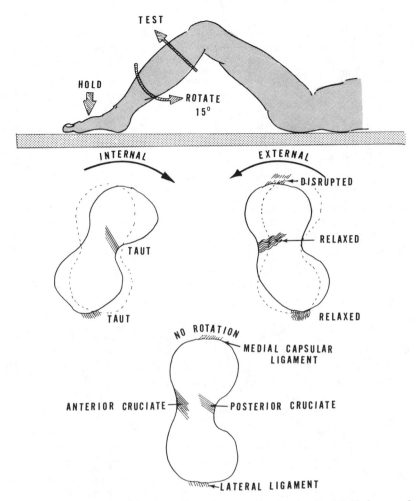

FIGURE 56. Rotatory instability test. Recumbent patient is examined with knee and hip flexed to 90°. Examiner sits on plantigrade foot (hold). Tibia is examined with 15° internal, no rotation, then 15° external rotation. The examiner pulls tibia forward upon the femur (test). With tibia *externally* rotated, the anterior cruciate ligament is relaxed as are the lateral ligaments. Excessive anterior displacement indicates medial capsular disruption (a "positive" test). With tibia *internally* rotated forward, movement of tibia upon femur is limited by posterolateral capsule, posterior cruciate ligament, fibular collateral ligament, and popliteus tendon and tensor fascia lata (not shown). With tibia *externally* rotated, the test is to determine adequacey of (1) medial capsular ligament, (2) anterior portion of medial collateral ligament, and (3) ultimately, the anterior cruciate ligament (if 1 and 2 are torn).

MODERATE SPRAIN. Swelling is noted locally. Frequently, some effusion of the joint occurs, which indicates excessive joint movement occurred at the time of injury. Pain can be elicited by stressing the joint, but normal movement may also be painful and physical limitation is self imposed. Locking may occur if there is concurrent meniscus injury or moderate

71

joint effusion or hemarthrosis. Instability can be ascertained if the involved joint is carefully compared with the opposite joint.

Treatment consists of complete resting of the knee by bedrest or a wheelchair with leg elevated and with ice packs. Any ambulation for personal needs requires crutches and *no* weight bearing on the involved leg. Ice packs are usually of value for the first 24 to 72 hours; with cessation of pain and effusion application of heat may be substituted. Pressure wrapping is valuable with the type and manner dependent on the expertise of the person treating the injury. An example of pressure wrapping is shown in Figure 57. The joint should be aspirated if effusion is moderate or marked and should be repeated if there is recurrence. Intra-articular steroids have little to offer but are advocated by some authorities as is the instillation of hyaluronidase. Weight bearing is definitely prohibited. Ultimately, an exercise program should be undertaken. Application of a cast (see Fig. 57) is advisable if there is severe pain, marked effusion, and apparent instability.

Repeated aspirations must be done when bloody fluid is retrieved. If the aspirated fluid is cloudy and yellowish, aspiration may be followed by instilling steroids.

The duration of conservative treatment is not an exact feature. Three weeks must be considered as minimal in a moderately severe ligamentous sprain. Exercises of an isometric type must be started early and gradually progress into the resistive types (see Chapter 3). Gentle flexion may be started early within the restrictive confines of the cast; then, usually within five days of the removal of the cast gentle flexion may be continued with greater range.

Persistence or aggravation of pain or effusion or both is an indication to decrease the intensity of the treatment program, especially the exercises and weight bearing. Re-examination at this stage may alter the classification of the degree of sprain.

SEVERE LIGAMENTOUS SPRAIN . This implies that the ligament is torn through its substance and away from its attachment with or without avulsing a piece of bone or cartilage. Disability is severe and immediate. Joint *instability* results. Swelling, if it occurs, is immediate and usually marked. Locking may occur because of a concommitent tear in a meniscus or because of the severity of the effusion. Early examination is of utmost importance before swelling, pain, and protective spasms obscure the picture. X-ray films with valgus or varus stress will reveal excessive motion of the joint of an unphysiologic degree.

There are cardinal factors related to ligamentous injuries of the knee that clarify the interpretation of the examination. Experimentally (Palmer), the knee with both cruciate ligaments removed remains laterally stable in the fully extended position; excessive rocking is possible however, with the knee slightly flexed. Removal of both collateral liga-

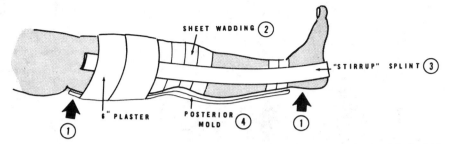

FIGURE 57. Method of pressure dressing and casting. The leg is held behind the thigh and the heel *(1)* to permit the tibia to hang, thus relaxing the anterior cruciate ligament. First wrap is sheet wadding (or gauze) *(2)* for uniform compression. A stirrup splint made of plaster strips *(3)* is used to prevent lateral motion. A posterior mold splint *(4)* with the foot dorsiflexed is then applied, and a final wrap around of gauze or 6 inches of a thin layer of plaster is used.

ments in an otherwise intact joint maintains knee stability in *hyperextension* but permits rocking with knee in slight flexion. Tear of the posterior capsule does not materially influence lateral stability. These findings imply that instability in the *hyperextended* knee position indicates damage to the cruciate ligaments and that lateral instability with the *knee flexed* indicates damage to the tibial collateral ligaments (Fig. 58).

Mere tear of the tibial collateral ligament does not cause joint lateral mobility in full extension and *no* drawer sign. With knee flexed to 90° and foot flexed by examiner, a *positive drawer sign* implies excessive motion of the tibia upon the femur on a horizontal anteroposterior motion as compared to the other (normal) side (Fig. 59). Tear of anterior cruciate only causes *no* lateral instability but permits an increased drawer effect and allows greater knee hyperextension. Tear of the anterior cruciate ligament *and* the tibial collateral ligament allows lateral instability that increases as the knee is flexed and allows a positive drawer sign. Lateral motion of 10 to 15° with knee fully extended is possible.

A knee injury in which external rotation occurs to the already flexed knee initiates a sequence of injury: (1) initial tearing of the deep medial ligament (capsule), (2) tearing of the tibial collateral ligament, and (3) tearing of the anterior cruciate ligament (Fig. 60).

In a severe injury, a blood effusion indicates damage to internal structures of the knee as well as to the ligaments. Tearing of the tibial ligament *without* synovial damage will not cause effusion, merely local edema and ecchymosis.

In treatment of severe ligamentous injuries with resultant instability, there are advocates of immediate surgery and advocates of prolonged conservative treatment. Experimentally, it has been shown that ligaments in which some fibers remain and in which there is good circulation regenerate well. With poor circulation, there is scar formation that is of poorer

73

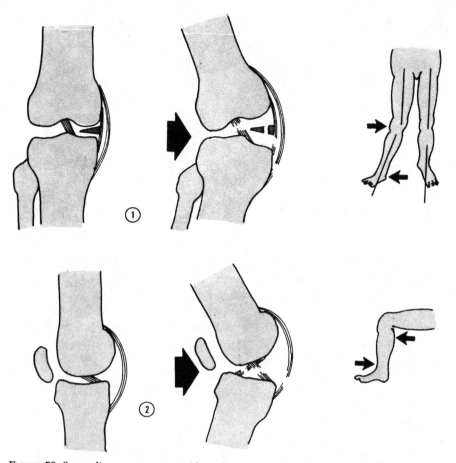

FIGURE 58. Severe ligamentous sprain (the unhappy triad). *1*, Lateral stress causing disruption of the medial collateral ligament, the medial meniscus, and the anterior cruciate ligament (the unhappy triad). *2*, Lateral view of a severe anterior stress causing hyperextension of the joint and disrupting both anterior and posterior cruciate ligaments and the posterior capsule. Clinically it has a positive drawer sign. *Far Right,* Arrows indicate the direction of movement by the examiner.

quality than ligamentous growth. Avulsion of the anterior cruciate ligament from it's femur attachment interferes with its blood supply and healing is poor; avulsion from its tibial attachment causes retraction and *no* healing.

In many cases, prolonged conservative treatment will result in a stable knee but of lesser stability than the early and adequately operated knee. Even in a knee with adequate surgical repair instability frequently results, especially when there is a concomittent meniscus or patellar injury, or both.

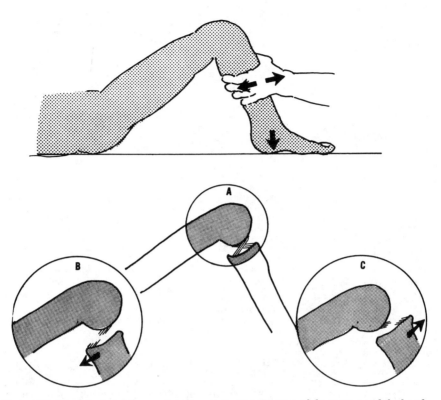

FIGURE 59. The drawer test for cruciate ligaments. *Top,* Position of the patient and the hands of the examiner in this test. The foot is fixed upon the examining table and the lower leg is horizontally moved proximally and distally. *Bottom, A,* The knee with intact cruciate ligaments that move a minimal distance equal to the opposite normal leg; *B,* Tear of the posterior cruciate with the tibia moving backward upon the femur; *C,* Movement elicited in a torn anterior cruciate. Excessive motion is possible in both directions if both cruciates are torn.

Careful consideration must be given the possibility of vascular or nerve injury when the ligamentous injuries are of significant severity to cause dislocation. The posterior popliteal artery is attached superiorly to the femur by the tendinous hiatus of the adductor magnus muscle and permits no mobility. The artery descends beneath the tendinous arch of the soleus and here it is firmly attached to the tibia. Hyperextension or shear dislocation of the knee in an anteroposterior direction can cause disruption of the artery. Lateral subluxation or severe varus injuries can damage the common peroneal nerve (Fig. 61). Conservative treatment of dislocation (Taylor et al.) has recently been claimed to give as good results as operative repair when there has been no vascular or nerve damage but merely ligamentous and capsular insult.

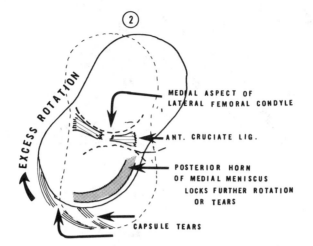

FIGURE 60. Sequence of ligamentous injury. In the flexed knee (to 90°), excessive external rotation results in tearing of the capsule (deep medial ligament). The tibial collateral ligament tears under the combination of abduction stress and further rotation, and ultimately the anterior cruciate ligament tears with further stress.

SUPERIOR TIBIOFIBULAR JOINT

Pain in the lateral aspect of the knee may occur due to pathology of the superior tibiofibular joint. Full understanding of this joint must be had before pathology and symptoms can be appreciated.

The fibula extends laterally the full length of the lower leg. At the ankle, it flares laterally to form the lateral malleolus of the ankle mortise. Superiorly, the fibula expands to form the fibular head. The inferior tibiofibular articulation is nonsynovial, whereas there is synovium in the superior joint. The head of the fibula articulates with the posterior inferior lateral aspect of the lateral tibial condyle in two possible manners. The articulation may be horizontal or oblique with the former having greater rotatory capability (Fig. 62).

As the knee flexes and extends (the femoral tibial articulation), there is simultaneous rotation (see Chapter 2); internal rotation with flexion and external rotation with extension. Thus, there must be tibial rotation. Ankle dorsiflexion and plantar flexion do not occur as isolated movements but also require tibial rotation. As the rotation occurs at different degrees at its superior and inferior aspect, the tibia and fibula rotate upon each other.

There are three movements between the tibia and the fibula (1) rotation, (2) anterior-posterior movement, and (3) superior-inferior movement. The primary function of the superior tibiofibular joint is to mini-

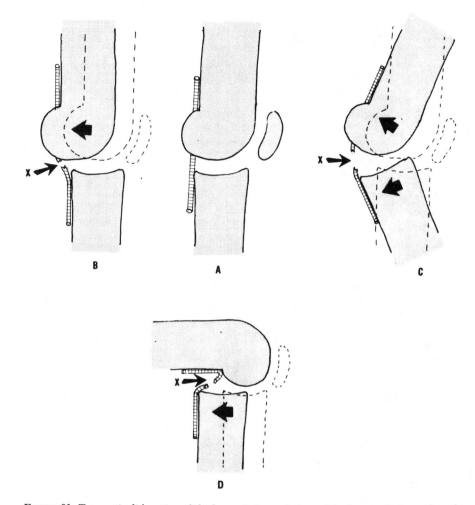

FIGURE 61. Traumatic dislocation of the knee. A, Lateral view of the knee with the popliteal artery adherent to the lower femur and the upper tibia; B, Direct injury to the femur, causing posterior luxation (shear) with arterial tear, (X). C, Hyperextension injury; D, Common auto accident injury with flexed knee, causing the tibia to dislocate posteriorly. Here also there is blood vessel injury.

mize torsional stresses at the ankle joint, decrease lateral tibial bending, and decrease weight-bearing torsion.

At the ankle, the anterior portion of the talus is wider than the posterior aspect, so ankle dorsiflexion separates the ankle mortise. The widening is restricted by the interosseous membrane. Widening can occur by the fibers that are normally oblique, becoming horizontal (Fig. 63). Separation of the tibia and the fibula ranges between 0.13 and 1.8 mm. If this

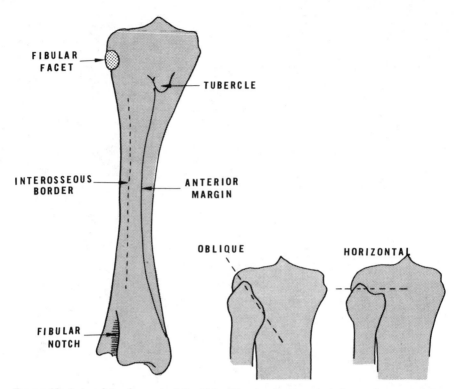

FIBULAR FACET

TUBERCLE

INTEROSSEOUS BORDER

ANTERIOR MARGIN

OBLIQUE

HORIZONTAL

FIBULAR NOTCH

FIGURE 62. Anteriolateral aspect of the tibia. The anterior margin is depicted to orient this aspect. The interosseous border is the site of attachment of the membrane fibers to the fibula. The fibular articulates with the facet and within the notch. The fibular joint with the facet may be oblique allowing mainly vertical movement or horizontal, allowing rotation.

occurs at the ankle mortise, it must also be dissipated at the superior tibiofibular articulation.

Injury Mechanisms

Pain, when present, is noted at the lateral or posterolateral aspect of the knee. Symptoms are annoying rather than disabling. Tenderness may be elicited by mobilization of the fibular tibial joint in an anterior posterior manner. The fibular head held between the examiner's thumb and index finger, then moved backward and forward, may elicit pain and tenderness. As the biceps femoris muscle attaches to the fibular head, resisted knee flexion with simultaneous rotation of the tibia may elicit pain. Weight bearing on the single affected leg with that knee slightly flexed has been specified as a provocative diagnostic test.

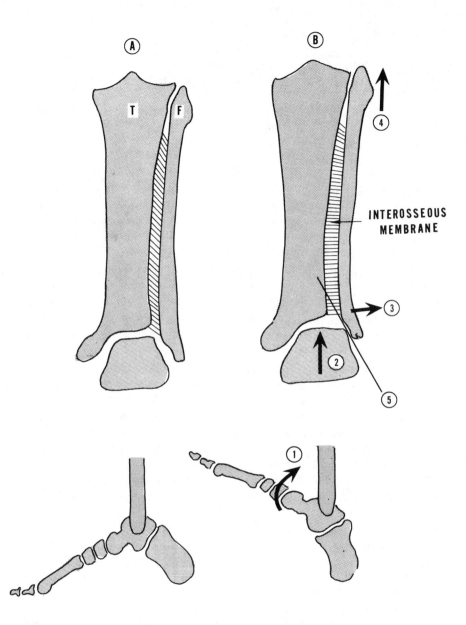

FIGURE 63. Fibular movement from ankle movement. A, Anterior view in the lower extremity with the ankle neutral showing the interosseous fibers being oblique. (B), As the ankle dorsiflexes (1), the anterior portion of the talus (2) separates the tibia (T) and fibula (3), causing the membrane fibers to become horizontal. The fibula also arises vertically (4) as it separates from the tiba. The oblique plane of the talus (5) mechanically separates the ankle mortise on weight bearing.

Treatment

Oral anti-inflammatory drugs may be effective as well as are local injections of an anesthetic agent with steroids. Local pressure dressing over the fibular head is of value.

If the joint has been dislocated, it can be easily reduced by external manipulation. This is done by placing the knee at 90° flexion then applying direct pressure upon the fibular head. An audible "pop" indicates reduction. This is then followed by immobilizing the knee in a walking cast including the foot and ankle for a period of three weeks.

Surgical repair is considered only in severe recurrent or persistent painful conditions. The procedures vary according to the experience of the surgeon and vary from capsular repair with postoperative casting to resection of the proximal fibula.

RUPTURE OF QUADRICEPS MECHANISM

Disruption of the quadriceps extensor mechanism may occur from direct and indirect trauma. Tear can occur in the muscle at the level of the muscle tendon junction, within the tendon, at the tendo-osseous junction of the upper or lower pole of the patella, within the tendon below the patella, or where the tendon attaches to the tibial tubercle.

Generally, direct trauma is caused by a forceful blow upon a contracted quadriceps muscle, usually when the knee is slightly flexed. It occurs more often in the aged or deconditioned individual. In the aged, the site of avulsion is mostly a separation of the tendon from the patella. In the young, the injury is usually from violent athletic activities and avulsion occurs mostly at the tendotubercle insertion.

The history is often that of an aged, overweight, and poorly conditioned individual who, descending stairs or jumping down, sustained a severe pain in the anterior knee area, felt or heard a snapping, and fell suddenly to the ground. Examination reveals swelling and tenderness at the site of tear. A sulcus may be palpable. There is inability to extend the knee, unless the tear is incomplete, in which case quadriceps power is present but diminished. Type of treatment is surgical repair of the tear followed by rehabilitation exercises.

Disruption of the tendon from the tubercle may occur from direct trauma but more often it is the result of indirect injury. Clinically, there is acute pain, local tenderness, probable swelling, and impaired knee extension. A gap is usually palpable and the patella, both palpably and by x-ray study, is situated higher than normal.

The indirect mechanism of injury requires some discussion. Injury to the extensor mechanism occurs in running when the foot is on the ground and the athlete is accelerating or decelerating, usually the latter. Forward motion is

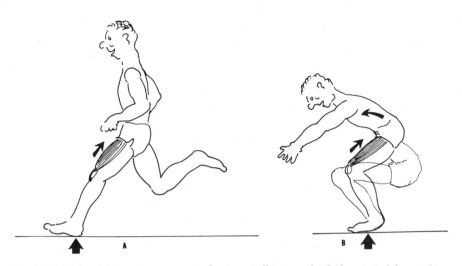

FIGURE 64. Indirect injury to extensor mechanism. A illustrates the decleration of the quadriceps during running at the time of leading foot strike with knee slightly bent; B reveals the acute stress of the quadriceps during the last phase of a jump.

decelerated at foot strike of the leading leg and the knee is bent more than during the similar phase of foot-heel strike in walking. Because running is essentially a series of coordinated jumps, the full body weight adds to the force of foot strikes (Fig. 64). In teenagers, the epiphysis and tendons are weaker than the muscle-tendon unions, thus injury is more apt to occur at this site.

Treatment of disruption in the young may merely require immobilization in a cast for one month but, when there is significant avulsion, surgical repair is desirable. Complications of extensor mechanism disruption by patellar dislocation or fracture will be discussed in a later chapter.

MYOSITIS OSSIFICANS

This condition is a frequent complication of contusion and hematoma caused by trauma to a muscle near its insertion to the bone. The implication that myositis is inflammation within the muscle is disputed. Rather it is considered to be periosteal in origin with the muscle avulsing the periosteum and causing a periosteal hematoma that invades the overlying muscle. There may actually be a small fragment of bone and periosteum that invades the muscle or invasion of periosteal cells into the overlying muscle hematoma, or a combination of both. The mass is considered pure bone directly attached to the adjacent bone or separated by a thin layer of muscle.

If rest is instituted after the trauma, the blood will usually be absorbed, but continued activity, further blows, unwise massage, and so forth may cause ultimate ossification. Early x-ray films usually are negative, thus

81

they should be repeated within three weeks if the mass persists. Treatment is conservative to prevent further bleeding and encourage absorption. Rest is mandatory. Ice applications should be followed within several days by heat. Massage if contraindicated. Gradually instituting gentle range of motion of the knee will minimize contracture and regain quadriceps strength. Rarely is surgery indicated, even in the well-ossified masses.

BIBLIOGRAPHY

ABBOTT, L, SAUNDERS, JD, BOST, FC, AND ANDERSON, C: *Injuries to ligaments of the knee.* J Bone Joint Surg 26-A:503, 1944.

BARNETT, CH AND NAPIER, JR: *The axis of rotation at the ankle joint in man: Its influence upon the talus and mobility of the fibula.* J Anat 86, 1952.

BENTLEY, G: *Chondromalacia patellae.* J Bone Joint Surg 52-A:221, 1970.

BETZ, RC, et al: *The percutaneous lateral retinacular release.* Orthopedics 5(1):57, 1982.

BLATZ, DJ, FLEMING, R, AND MCCARROLL, J: *Suprapatellar plica: A study of their occurence and role in internal derangement of the knee in active duty personnel.* Orthopedics 4(2):181, February 1981.

CAILLIET, R: *Foot and Ankle Pain,* ed 2. FA Davis, Philadelphia, 1983.

CLOSE, JR AND INMAN, V: *The action of the ankle joint.* University of California, Berkley, Series 11, Issue 22, 1952.

DE ANDRADE, JR, GRANT, C, AND ST J DIXON, A: *Joint distension and reflex muscle inhibition in the knee.* J Bone Joint Surg 47-A(2):313, 1965.

DEVAS, M AND GALSKI, A: *Treatment of chondromalacia patellae by transposition of the tibial tubercle.* Br Med J 1:589, 1973.

EYRING, EJ AND MURRAY, WR: *The effect of joint position on the pressure of intra-articular effusion.* J Bone Joint Surg 46-A(6):1235, September 1964.

GOODFELLOW, J, HUNGERFORD, DS, AND WOODS, C: *Patello-femoral joint mechanics and pathology. 2. Chondromalacia patellae.* J Bone Joint Surg 58-B(3):291, 1976.

GOODFELLOW, J, HUNGERFORD, DS, AND ZINDEL, M: *Patello-femoral joint mechanics and pathology. 1. Functional anatomy of the patello-femoral joint.* J Bone Joint Surg 58-B(3):287, 1976.

HARRISON, R AND HIDENACH, JC: *Dislocation of the upper end of the fibula.* J Bone Joint Surg 41-B, 1959.

INSALL, J: *Current concepts review of patellae pain.* J Bone Joint Surg 64-A(1):147, 1982.

KENNEDY, JC AND FOWLER, PJ: *Medial and anterior instability of the knee. An anatomical and clinical study using stress machines.* J Bone Joint Surg 53-A:1257, 1971.

KENNEDY, JC, WEINBERG, HW, AND WILSON, AS: *The anatomy and function of the anterior cruciate.* J Bone Joint Surg 56-A(2):223, 1974.

MAQUET, P: *Mechanics and osteoarthritis of the patellofemoral joint.* Clin Orthop 144:70, 1979.

MERCHANT, AC: *Isolated patellofemoral arthritis: Its significance and treatment.* Contemporary Orthopedics Vol 3,II:1015, 1981.

MERCHANT, AC, ET AL: *Roentgenographic analysis of patellofemoral congruence.* J Bone Joint Surg 56-A(7):1391, 1974.

MEYERS, MH AND HARVEY, JP, JR: *Traumatic dislocation of the knee joint. A study of eighteen cases.* J Bone Joint Surg 53-A:16, 1971.

O'DONOGHUE, DH: *Treatment of Injuries to Athletes.* WB Saunders, Philadelphia, 1962.

O'DONOGHUE, DH: *Surgical treatment of fresh injuries to the major ligaments of the knee.* J Bone Joint Surg 32-A:721, 1950.

OGDEN, JA: *The anatomy and function of the proximal tibiofibular joint.* Clin Orthop 101:186, 1974.

OUTERBRIDGE, RE: *The etiology of chondromalacia patellae.* J Bone Joint Surg 43-B(4):752, 1961.

OUTERBRIDGE, RE: *Further studies on the etiology of chondromalacia patellae.* J Bone Joint Surg 46-B:179, 1964.

OWRE, A: *Condromalacia patellae.* Acta Chir Scand (Suppl):41, 1936.

PALMER, L: *On the injuries of the ligaments of the knee joints. A clinical study.* Acta Chir Scand (Suppl):53, 1938.

PIPKIN, G: *Knee injuries: The role of the suprapatellar plica and suprapatellar bursa in simulating internal derangement.* Clin Orthop 74:161, January 1971.

REYNOLDS, FC: *Injuries to ligaments of the knee.* Journal of the Omaha Mid-West Clinical Society 23:103, 1962.

SLOCUM, DB AND LARSON, RL: *Pes anserinus transplantation: A surgical procedure for control of the rotatory instability of the knee.* J Bone Joint Surg 50-A: 226, 1968.

SLOCUM, DB AND LARSON, RL: *Rotatory instability of the knee.* J Bone Joint Surg 50-A(2):211, March 1968.

SLOCUM, DB AND LARSON, RL: *Indirect injuries to the extensor mechanism of the knee in athletes.* Am J Orthop 6:248, 1964.

SMILLIE, JS: *Injuries of the Knee Joint,* ed 2. Livingston, Edinburgh, 1951.

TAYLOR, AR, ARDEN, GP, AND RAINEY, HA: *Traumatic dislocation of the knee.* J Bone Surg 54-B: 96, 1972.

WIBERG, G: *Roentgenographic and anatomic studies of the femoropatellar joint.* Acta Ortho Scand 12:319, 1941.

WILES, P, ANDREWS, PS, AND DEVAS, MB: *Chondromalacia of the patella.* J Bone Joint Surg 38-B:95, 1956.

83

CHAPTER 5

Patellar Injuries and Diseases

Injuries and diseases of the patella, which can impair this portion of the extensor mechanism of the knee, are so numerous that the subject merits separate consideration. In differentiating *injury* from *disease* it will be apparent that injury is considered as an important aspect of all patellar dysfunctions.

PATELLOFEMORAL ARTHRALGIA

Of the two knee joints, femorotibial and patellofemoral, the latter has been overlooked for many decades until recently. Pathology of this joint causes a large percentage of pain and disability of the knee, yet it is claimed that only one book solely regarding the patellofemoral joint has been written in English and that in 1977. Pathology of the patellofemoral joint other than fracture or dislocation is that of patellofemoral arthritis. Arthritis must be classified as resulting from excessive or abnormal stress, trauma, or from disease such as gout, infection, or rheumatoid arthritis that, albeit a systemic disease, predisposes the patellofemoral joint to isolated disease or impairment.

The normal mechanics of the patellofemoral joint are undergoing intensive study. This joint sustains the force of the most powerful muscle (quadriceps femoris) of the body, via a long lever arm (femur) and acts mechanically as a sesamoid bone to give mechanic leverage of a parallelogram to the knee joint (Fig. 65). The patellofemoral articulation contains the thickest hyaline cartilage of the body joints. It has been estimated that in the act of doing a deep knee bend, a pressure of seven times body weight is exerted upon this joint.

The patella has asymmetrical facets separated by a central ridge. The medial facet is larger than the lateral and each facettal plane is divided into three planes (Fig. 66). The patella articulates (tracts) within the concavity of the femoral condyles. As the tibiofemoral joint rotates about

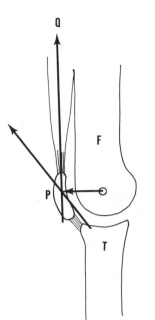

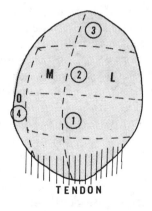

FIGURE 65. Parallelogram of knee joint. Parallelogram of force from quadriceps *(Q)* action through patella *(P)*, a sesamoid bone that angles force from femoral *(F)* alignment to attach to and extend the tibia *(T)*.

FIGURE 66. Facets of patella. The cartilaginous surface of the patella has a broader lateral *(L)* facet than the medial *(M)*. Each half *(M-L)* is divided into three facets with the inferior facet attaching the infrapatellar tendon. The bottom drawing depicts the medial *(M)*, lateral *(L)*, and odd *(O)* facets from a superior view.

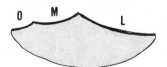

85

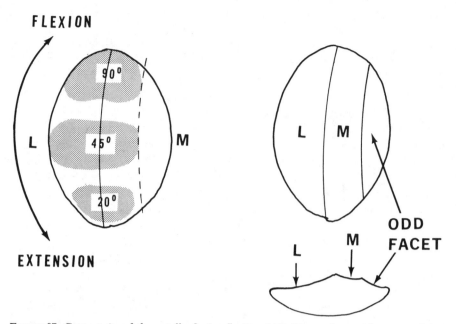

FLEXION

90°

L 45° M

20°

EXTENSION

L M

ODD

M FACET

L

FIGURE 67. Contact site of the patella during flexion. *Left,* Sites and area of contact of the patella to the femoral condyles during flexion of 20, 45, and 90°. The lateral *(L)* facets make contact through entire flexion-extension with no contact with the medial *(M)* or odd facets during physiologic tracting.

a vertical axis during flexion and extension of the knee joint (approximately 10°), the patella moves *with* the femur causing no displacement (Figs. 67 and 68).

Damage to the patellofemoral joint can be from a force overload or asymmetry of the articulation components. Early recognition and, hopefully, correction of these damaging components are evidently required as cartilage has limited regeneration possibilities once it has undergone degenerative changes. The force upon the patella is that of the quadriceps femoris group that inserts its pull at an angle—currently termed the "Q" angle. This angular pull applies asymmetrical patella tracting that when limited is physiologically accepted. The length of the infrapatellar ligament modifies the direction, angulation, and force of the quadriceps mechanics—the depth of the femoral condyles, protrusion of the patellar spine, and the symmetry of the patellar facets all influence the adequacy of the articular mechanics. The ligaments that attach to the patella insure its security or its instability (Fig. 69).

The patellofemoral joint is frequently overlooked as a site of pain, yet is a frequent region for pain production. To call all pain in the patellar region "chondromalacia patellae" is simplistic and misleading. Patellar pain implies pain from the bone itself, rather than from the usually impaired joint function. It would be better to call this knee pain patellofemoral arthralgia. There are numerous causes of patellofemoral pain that require discussion. These currently include (1) chondromalacia, (2) patellofemoral degenerative arthritis or basal degeneration, (3) fracture of the patella or osteochondral fracture, and (4) osteochondritis.

There are numerous causes of patellar cartilage damage that can be termed (1) overuse syndrome of normal cartilage, (2) malalignment with or without subluxation or dislocation, or (3) quadriceps abnormality (termed quadriceps dysplasia). Malalignment is simultaneously called "abnormal patellar tracting" in which there exists mechanical malfunction of the patellofemoral joint. The diagnosis of patellofemoral arthralgia requires careful evaluation of the specific mechanical cause of pain to insure proper correction of the offending factors.

Chondromalacia

Chondromalacia has become well established in regard to pathoanatomic changes of the articular cartilage. Three stages are established, (I) swelling and softening of the cartilage with no interruption of structure, (II) fissuring of the softened portion of the cartilage and, (III) the surface deforms in a manner termed fasciculation. Any later stage implies damage to cartilage with erosion and exposure of subchondral bone, better termed osteoarthritis. The changes in chrondromalacia are limited to the patellar cartilage (Stages I to III). When there is further damage as in Stage IV (osteoarthritis), damage is noted in the femoral cartilage.

Changes in the patellae cartilage are normally noted most often in people who reach middle age without symptoms or disability. If there has been malalignment with impaired "tracting," pain can result but not necessarily with changes in the cartilage. The exact cause of pain is not fully understood as there may be pain without chondromalacia in malalignment and pain with chondromalacia with normal tracting. *The current belief is that the cartilage changes are not the cause of patellofemoral pain but rather it is the pressure induced by abnormal patellar tracting that causes symptoms* (Fig. 70). It must be noted, however, that certain symptomatic patients have been relieved by correction or removal of the damaged cartilage.

Chondromalacia is a condition of adolescents or young adults, but is occurring with increasing severity and frequency in an older age group who take up jogging or running. There is no sexual relationship. Femoral patellar pain, other than degenerative arthritis or following direct trauma to the knee cap, is infrequent after the fourth decade of life. Chondromalacia, when found in the aging population is often, if not usually asymptomatic. Chondromalacia arthralgia conversely can be symptomatic *without* cartilage abnormality.

87

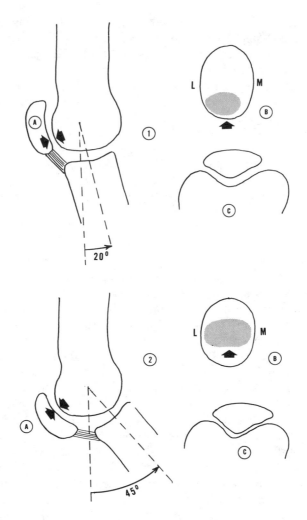

Goodfellow and colleagues have described the articular pathology of the patella. The normal wear and tear of joint articular cartilage has been well documented (Fig. 71). These changes occur from mechanical trauma and are age related, that is, expected as patients age. This is a surface degeneration with gradual "flaking" of the surface progressing to fibrillation and fissuring (Fig. 72). Ultimately, the cartilage is denuded in areas that expose subchondral bone and degenerative arthritis results. These changes gradually are noted in most patellae but need not cause symptoms until the later change of degenerative disease condition is noted in all aging patellae, most of which are asymptomatic but is not considered a source

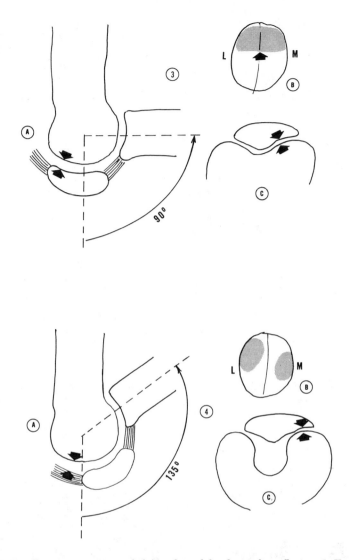

FIGURE 68. Patellar contact areas with femoral condyles during knee flexion. *1,* Knee flexed 20°: *A,* Lateral view of patellofemoral joint. *Arrows* depict site of contact. *B,* Area of contact of the patella *(shaded area)* (L = lateral, M = medial). *C,* Superior view showing patella within femoral condyles. At 20° flexion, there is contact symmetrically of the lateral and medial condyles to the patellar facets. Note, there is minimal or no pressure upon medial condyle. *2,* Knee flexed 45°: Pressure site upon patella in broader central zone *(C).* As in *1,* there is symmetrical pressure of medial and lateral patellar facets. *3,* Knee flexed 90°: The patellar contact is broad contact of the superior area of medial and lateral facets *(B).* In *C,* there is beginning to be more contact of medial facets. *4,* Knee flexed 135° (full flexion): The patellar facets contact both femoral condyles and the patella shifts *(C)* so that the odd facet contacts the medial condyle more firmly.

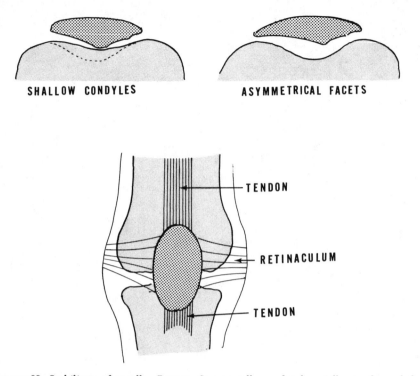

SHALLOW CONDYLES   ASYMMETRICAL FACETS

TENDON

RETINACULUM

TENDON

FIGURE 69. Stabilizers of patella. *Bottom*, Suprapatellar and infrapatellar tendons of the quadriceps mechanism. The retinaculum holds the patella in its central "tract." *Top*, Two conditions that permit the patella to sublux.

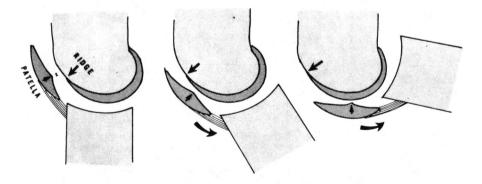

FIGURE 70. Mechanism of chondromalacia caused by the femoral condylar ridge. As the knee flexes, the patella is dragged across the ridge and irritates the patellar cartilage. The irritation occurs between 15 and 30° of flexion.

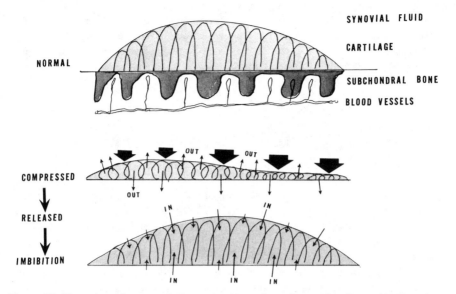

FIGURE 71. Normal cartilage metabolism. *Top,* Normal cartilage with collagen fibrills within matrix upon subchondral bone (schematic), nutrition comes from influx of synovial fluid and dialysate of bone blood vessels. *Middle,* Pressure exudes hyaluronidase, mucin, chondroitin sulphate, and so forth from cartilage into synovial cavity and into bone blood vessels. *Bottom,* Imbibition of nutrient fluids from release of compression of cartilage.

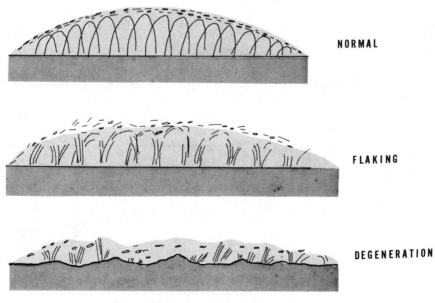

FIGURE 72. Stages of degenerative arthritis.

91

of patellofemoral pain in the young. This form of cartilage degeneration is noted most often in the *odd* facet surface. Only in later life, when degenerative arthritis has developed, that is, subchondral bone exposure, do symptoms occur.

Basal Degeneration

Contrary to the age related surface degnerative changes that have been described, a condition of *basal* degeneration has been noted in arthrotomies of symptomatic patients. Basal degeneration occurs in the *deep* portion of the cartilage sparing the surface. The first stage of basal degneration is fasciculation of the collagen fibers, that is, bunching of the fibers. This occurs in a small segment with all the adjacent fibers remaining intact. The distal portion of the fascicles deteriorate and fragment forming a "blister" that ruptures causing a fissure from the surface to the subchondral bone.

Basal degeneration is not the primary nor the inclusive cause of patellofemoral arthralgias in adolescents or young adults, but is found in some at arthrotomy or arthroscopy. It has been reported in asymptomatic knees as well as absent in symptomatic knees. It is, however, one of the causes of chondromalacia patellae and when found requires special treatment. As will be discussed later, one of the accepted treatments of chondromalacia patellae is to shave the cartilage. With basal degeneration, the choice would be to *exercise* the localized area of degeneration leaving the surrounding normal cartilage intact.

As the site of basal degeneration is at the ridge between the odd facet and the medial facets (See Fig. 67), this is the site of maximum pressure when the knee is flexed to 90° as in the sitting position. This knee-flexed, painful position is characteristic of chondromalacia patellae in young adults. Classically, pain is felt in the region of the kneecap when the knee is flexed and weight bearing. Patients complain of pain ascending or descending stairs, especially the latter (Fig. 73). Prolonged sitting with knee fully flexed may cause pain, slightly aggravated by the movement of "getting up," but relieved by fully extending the knee. Crepitation may be experienced and can be elicited by the examiner. This sound is frequently heard in pain-free knees and is not related to the severity of the cartilage damage when it is associated with patellofemoral pain (Fig. 74).

Examination reveals the reproduction of the pain by pressure upon the patella with the knee extended, then movement of the patella distally and proximally (Fig. 75). With the knee extended and the quadriceps relaxed, the patella can be medially and laterally moved and the under surface (medial) of the patella can be palpated.

Effusion is rare as is joint limitation. Usually both knees may be affected but unilateral patellofemoral pain is noted. Spontaneous recovery

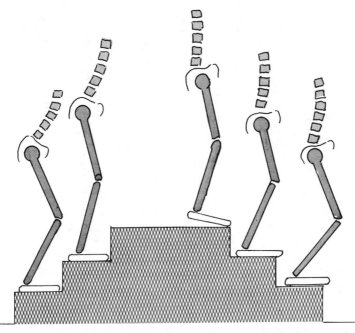

FIGURE 73. Knee in stair climbing and descending. As the person climbs the stairs, the knee flexes approximately 50° and the body leans forward; in descending, the body remains more erect above the hip joint with knee flexing to approximately 65°.

may occur but some progress to the degenerative arthritic phase. The patient occasionally complains of the knee "giving way" or catching with "clicking." Locking occurs.

The examination must evaluate the tracing of the patella. These may be:

1. increase in quadriceps angle "Q"
2. laxity of the quadriceps tendon due to genu recurvatum
3. a shallow patellar fossa
4. abnormal inferior patellar contour
5. marked internal femoral torsion
6. excessive tibial torsion
7. patella alta
8. severe foot pronation
9. secondary to internal femorotibial damage such as meniscal disease
10. cruciate ligament instability, collateral ligament laxity, or paretic vastus medialis muscle.

Any or all of these may be present as well as other conditions such as genu varus or genu valgus.

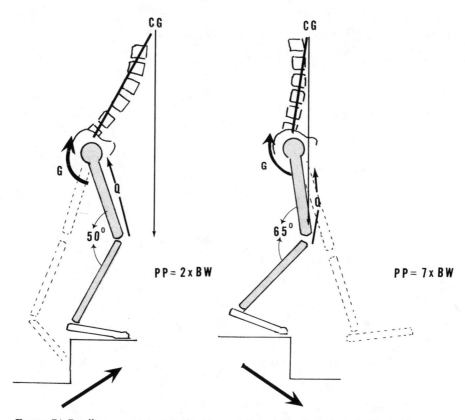

FIGURE 74. Patellar pressure in stair climbing and descending. *Left*, Stair climbing. The knee flexes an average of 50°, the body leans forward advancing the center of gravity *(CG)* and increases the gluteal efficiency *(G)*. The patellar pressure *(PP)* due to quadriceps contracture *(Q)* is two times body weight *(BW)*. *Right*, Stair descending. The knee flexes an average of 65°, the body reclines backward of center of gravity, gluteal efficiency is decreased and patellar pressure is seven times body weight. This is one of the factors resulting in patellar pain (chondromalacia).

Basal degeneration can only be ascertained by surgical exploration. A blunt probe will reveal a small area of softening around which all the cartilage remain normal. As the degeneration progresses, the surface cartilage bulges then disrupts allowing cartilage debris to erupt into the joint.

Radiologic Evaluation

Radiologic views of the femorotibial and patellofemoral joints may confirm the clinical impression or reveal pathology not evident clinically. Radiologic views of the patellofemoral articulation require special axial

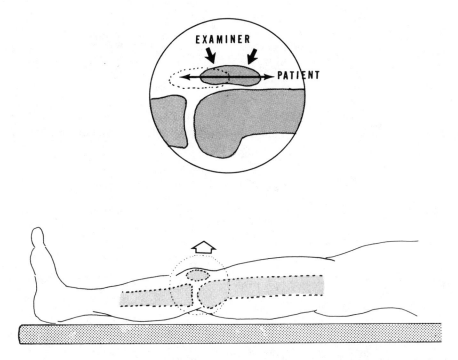

FIGURE 75. Examination for patellofemoral articulation. With leg extended and quadriceps relaxed, the examiner presses down upon the patella in a downward then upward direction. The patient then slowly contracts and relaxes the quadriceps, pain and crepitation may be elicited.

views. There are standard axial views as well as newer techniques (Fig. 76). Arthrograms are not usually diagnostic. Arthroscopy is of value to reveal the appearance of the cartilage but not always valuable to determine patellofemoral incongruence.

Treatment

Patellofemoral arthralgia should always be treated conservatively. The presence of loose bodies within the joint is the exception. Treatment is essentially nonpainful isometric exercises (Fig. 77) and patellar bracing. The exercises are:

1. Full extension of the affected leg with elevation of the patella—"tightening the knee"—which essentially contracts the quadriceps isometrically and brings the patella up upon the femur. This is done gently and slowly *without pain*. The opposite knee is flexed to protect the low back during exercises.

95

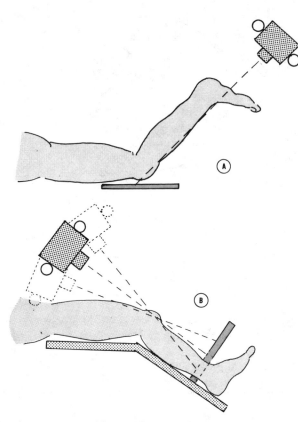

FIGURE 76. A technique suggested by Merchant (A) is claimed to be more accurate than the standard axial views taken at 45° knee flexion, then 30 and 60° (B).

2. The extended leg is slowly elevated against the resistance of a weight at the ankle. Weights may vary from 2 to 15 lbs depending on the age of the patient and the strength of the quadriceps.
3. The leg is extended to 45°, held for approximately five seconds, then slowly lowered.
4. The leg is relaxed then the exercise is resumed—gradually, 15 to 50 repetitions are desirable each session with three to five sessions daily.

A subsequent exercise then is added if tolerated by the patient, that is, causes no discomfort. The patient in the supine position with opposite hip and knee flexed, has the knee in a 15 to 20° flexion with a rolled towel beneath the knee. With the foot or ankle weight in place, the knee is slowly extended—held briefly and slowly returned to the flexed position, then rested. This exercise strengthens the knee extensors within the last 10 to 15° of extension and presumably exercises the vastus medialis.

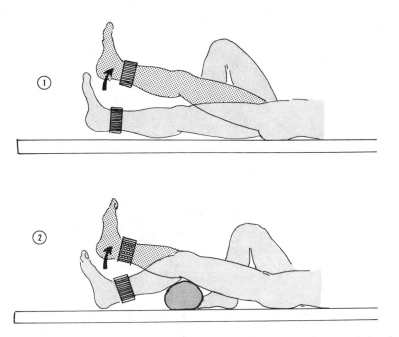

FIGURE 77. Quadriceps exercise for chondromalacia patella. *1*, With leg extended and re-laxed, the quadriceps is gently "tightened," the leg is lifted slowly to 45°—held there briefly then lowered—once down, the quadriceps is relaxed. The opposite leg is flexed to "protect" the low back. *2*, The involved leg is flexed approximately 45° with a weight about the ankle (2 lb to gradually 10 to 15 lb). The leg is slowly extended—held—then slowly relaxed. Both *1* and *2* are done with 20 repetitions 3 to 5 times daily.

The basis for pain relief from these exercises is far from documented. It is conceivable that the alternating compression and relaxation of the carti-lage *without* shearing forces enhances inhibition of fluid within the carti-lage and regains more normal tissue. When there has been abrasion of the cartilage, in osteoarthritis, this explanation may not be acceptable. Strengthening the vastus medialis may assist in realigning and stabilizing the patella in its femoral tract. Lateral deviation of the patella is consid-ered a major incongruence of the articulation. The hamstrings must also be strengthened. This is done in the prone position through a short arc: from knee pull straight to 30° flexion—gradually increasing to 20 to 40 repetitions: one leg at a time (Fig. 78).

A brace to restrain lateral or medial movement of the patella may be of value. This brace is elastic, thus allowing some flexion of the knee. It incorporates a horseshoe-shaped pad that encircles the patella to permit ascension and descension, but limits lateral and medial movements.

When malalignment is severe, surgical correction may be indicated. These malalignments include excessive quadriceps angle, lateral patellar

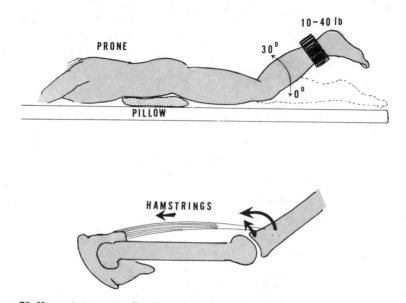

FIGURE 78. Hamstring exercise. *Top*, Patient is prone with pillow under abdomen to decrease lordosis. Knee flexes slowly from full extension (0°) to 30° beginning with 10 lb increasing to 40 lb, repeating exercise 30 times each series. *Bottom*, The hamstrings flex the knee and lightly shear the tibia posteriorly.

tracting, patella alba, or significant patellar incongruence. *Lateral release* of the retinaculum is the easiest to perform and reportedly the most effective. The lateral retinaculum and fibers of the vastus lateralis are released to allow the patella to move medially. The *vastus medialis* muscle *insertion* upon the patella can be advanced, thus bringing the patella more medially without altering the quadriceps angle in the length of the patella tendon. This procedure may be combined with a lateral release. The medius advancement is a more formidable procedure and should be considered only in severe intractible conditions.

The Hauser procedure, tibial *tubercle transfer,* is no longer widely used as there is reported later osteoarthritic changes within the patellofemoral joint. As described by Maquet, the *tibial tubercle* is *elevated* by at least 2 cm. This separates the patella from the femoral condyle and has been reasonably successful but more so in severe osteoarthritis than in chondromalacia patellae.

PATELLAR SHAVING. Shaving the patella has regained favor with the advent of arthroscopy. When there is marked irregularity of the patellar cartilage shaving, this damaged tissue restores smoothness of articular surface. The cartilage is replaced by fibrocartilage and the procedure allegedly does not cause prolonged debility as it must, to be successful, be followed by immediate motion and exercises. Shaving procedures are usually combined with realignment procedures. In the presence of basal chondromalacia, when found via arthroscope or arthrotomy, excision of the bleb rather than shaving is recommended.

In severe patellofemoral degenerative arthritis, patellar replacement has been advocated but this is a salvage procedure that has, thus far, limited success. Patellectomy is probably preferred in severe intractable patellofemoral pain and disability but its success in relieving pain is not guaranteed and most often results in quadriceps weakness and knee instability.

PATELLAR DISLOCATION

In normal motion of gliding in the patellar groove of the distal anterior aspect of the femur, the patella is dependent upon the tendinous aspect of the quadriceps mechanism, the depth of the groove, its own intrinsic structure, and the alignment of the entire musculoskeletal components of the lower extremity (Fig. 79).

In review of anatomy, the patella has a smooth posterior articulating surface that is covered with cartilage and presents two facets divided by a vertical ridge that fits into a corresponding groove between the two condyles of the femur.

Dislocation in which the patella leaves its femoropatellar groove can occur for various reasons. An acute injury or violent stress can cause dislocation of an otherwise normal patella. Such insults occur from severe falls or external injuries, such as automobile accidents or athletic injuries with violent lateral rotatory stress imposed upon the knee on the weight-bearing leg.

Dislocation can be present in the newborn as a congenital abnormality. The patella may be poorly formed, the femoropatellar groove inadequate, or the alignment faculty because of severe varus or valgus knee. Diagnosis in the newborn usually is made by clinical examination because x-ray film of the knee fails to reveal the patella, which does not ossify until ages two to six. Correction of the genu valgus is usually considered in the newborn.

Recurrent Dislocation

An acute dislocation can predispose the knee to further episodes. Other factors can exist that predispose dislocation from minor stress upon the knee (Fig. 80). These include:

1. Marked genu valgum that laterally displaces the patella or improperly aligns the extensor mechanism.
2. An elongated patellar tendon that causes a slack in the patellofemoral junction.

99

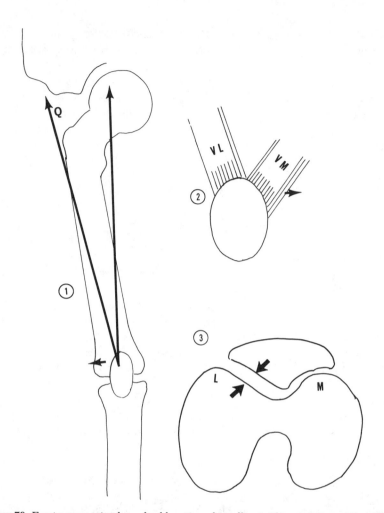

FIGURE 79. Forces preventing lateral subluxation of patella. *1*, The quadriceps *(Q)* pull from patella to anterior superior. Iliac crest is at an angle from the line of the femur, this angle is termed Q angle. *2*, The vastus lateralis *(VL)* pulls the patella superiorly and laterally, the vastus medialis *(VM)* neutralizes this by pulling patella medially (arrow). *3*, Superior view of patellofemoral joint showing the seating of the patella with the anterior femoral condyles. Lateral *(L)* prevents lateral deviation, medial condyle *(M)* does not protrude to same extent.

3. A deficient vastus medialis.
4. External tibial torsion.
5. A shallow patellar groove on the femur.
6. A lateral patellar attachment on the tubercle.
7. A shallow lateral femoral condyle.
8. A deformed patella.

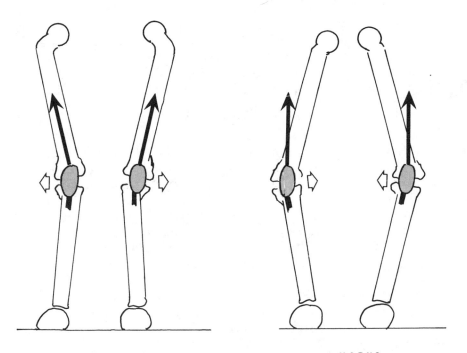

GENU VALGUS   GENU VARUS

FIGURE 80. Mechanism of patellar dislocation. There is lateral deviation of the patella in genu valgus and medial deviation in genu varus *(open arrows)*, tibial or femoral rotation intensify the stress.

One of the first symptoms is a tendency for the knee to buckle, causing the patient to fall or lose balance. Pain and tenderness over the anterior knee area follows. Effusion is frequent but is not as severe as in an internal knee injury. There may be some difficulty in extending the knee but when extension is accomplished, either actively or passively, the patella returns to its normal position.

Examination reveals one or more of the contributing factors listed. There is usually excessive laxity of the extensor mechanism and excessive movement of the patella is possible generally in a lateral direction. The vastus medialis may be atrophic. Crepitation is felt and heard between the patella and its femoral groove. X-ray studies in the adult may reveal a malformed patella, a shallow femoral condyle, or merely a faulty position of the patella as compared to the normal side. In cases of recurrent dislocation, chondromalacia patellae may be evident.

A recurrent dislocating patella frequently occurs as an associated condition of other knee joint pathology that impairs the extensor mechanism, such as the narrowing of the knee joint space, malalignment from meniscus disease, or degenerative arthritis.

There are many types of treatment advocated, evidence that no one form of treatment has proved to be completely effective. Repair is aimed at changing the line of quadriceps pull, restoring the depth of the femoral sulcus, or decreasing the quadriceps laxity. In severe patellar dislocation in which the paripatellar reticulum is torn, surgical repair is indicated.

PATELLAR FRACTURE

Fracture is frequent because of the exposed position of the patella and the severe stress imposed upon it in violent activites. Trauma is thus direct or indirect. Diagnosis should pose no problem if a fractured condition is suspected. The history may include a blow to the knee or a fall upon the patella (direct). In older, usually obese and deconditioned individuals, indirect injury is elicited by a history of a jump, descending the stairs, a forceful squat, and so forth with an audible and painful snap followed by a fall or loss of balance. Usually, the patient then is unable to extend the knee.

Examination reveals swelling about the patella, tenderness, and usually some effusion. The appearance of the patella may reveal deformity and occasionally fragments of the patella may be movable manually by the examiner. X-ray films are helpful in diagnosis.

Treatment may present problems but a cardinal rule exists: *the patella must be conserved if at all possible.* The concept that the patella is of no value to knee extensor function is not tenable. Excision of the patella is considered only when there has been severe comminution leaving no single fragment of significant size to be of value to the extensor mechanism.

Therefore, treatment may be conservative or surgical. In the conservative approach, effusion, and especially hemarthrosis, must be aspirated, repeatedly if necessary. A posterior mold splint that fully extends the knee is applied and the knee is packed in ice for several days until all swelling is eliminated. Then a skin-tight cast is applied, and replaced as needed to maintain firm contact, for a period of four to eight weeks. Crutch walking is permitted. Quadriceps setting exercises are begun early and carefully supervised to secure maintenance of quadriceps strength.

Surgical intervention requires good judgment by an experienced orthopedic surgeon. Surgery involves:

1. Replacement and fixation of the fragments.
2. Removal of entire patellar fragments. (Total or partial patellectomy as treatment of patellar fractures has resulted in good functional recovery with no adverse effect on knee motion, strength, or stability (Mishra). Complete excision is not usually followed by femoral condyle arthritic change nor ossification of the patellar tendon.)

102

3. Removal of all fragments, leaving only an adequate large fragment.
4. Replacement of the patella with a prosthesis.

Realignment of fragments with fixation is usually unsuccessful because congruity of the articular surface is not attainable and cannot be maintained against the forceful traction of the quadriceps and the poor osteogenesis of the patella. Nonunion of fragments or chondromalacia patellae is a fragment result. Good results from internal fixation usually exist when there are two equal fragments that approximate anatomically. Best results are reported when one large fragment can be salvaged and all other fragments removed.

Osteochondral fractures must be considered when x-ray studies fail to reveal any abnormality but clinical suspicion exists and when the history and symptoms are similar to that of a patellar fracture.

The history is usually of a teenager or young adult who sustains direct or indirect trauma, that is caused by twisting or jumping on a flexed, weight-bearing knee, thus giving rise to a lateral dislocation of the patella. An osteochondral fracture may result with or without a resultant loose body. Medial tenderness is elicited and the hemarthrosis may reveal flecks of fat in the aspirated fluid. X-ray films may reveal the loose body. Arthrography (see Chapter 3) may be necessary for diagnosis and, if available, should precede diagnostic arthrotomy.

Conservative treatment as mentioned in fractures is indicated, but surgical exploration is valid when symptoms are persistent or of greater severity than expected from physical examination and x-ray studies.

OSTEOCHONDRITIS

Osgood-Schlatter's Disease

This condition is osteochondritis of the tibial tubercle. It is observed in adolescents, usually boys, and frequently is bilateral. The onset is insidious. The patient is aware of pain and tenderness over the tibial tubercle. The condition is aggravated by exercise or from direct pressure such as kneeling. Swelling of the tubercle or the tendon where it attaches to the tubercle is noted.

During adolescence, the attachment of the tubercle to the tibial shaft is a weak link of the quadriceps mechanism. Repeated traction stresses predispose to minor avulsion of the ossification center. These changes are similar to those described in Larsen-Johannson's disease of the patella.

A theory has been postulated that bony changes are actually secondary to swelling, hemorrhage, and degenerative changes of the patellar tendon near its attachment. These changes in the tendon impair the circulation of

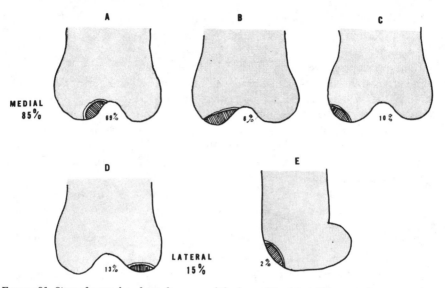

FIGURE 81. Sites of osteochondritis dissecans of the knee. *Top*, Most (85 percent) occur on the medial femoral condyle; *A*, Classical with 69 percent on the lateral border of the medial condyle; *B*, Extended classical with 6 percent; *C*, An inferiocentral site with 10 percent. *Bottom*, 15 percent occur on the lateral condyle; *D*, inferiocentral with 13 percent; *E*, An anterior site with 2 percent.

the underlying bone and cause irregular ossification. The ossification irregularities appear months after subsistence of the tendon swelling. Nature repairs the irregularity years after the onset.

The only abnormality noted clinically is swelling of the patellar tendon and some swelling of the tubercle with tenderness on pressure and from resisted quadriceps contraction. X-ray studies are negative early in the disease.

Usually, treatment is merely avoidance of excessive activity such as running and jumping, knee flexion, and kneeling. If the condition is more severe a cylindrical cast may be applied to the extended knee for several weeks to two months. Rarely is surgery considered. Such surgery consists of tendon splitting, multiple drilling of the tubercle, or bone grafting.

Larsen-Johannson's Disease

This is an osteochondritis condition affecting the poles of the patella, most often the inferior pole. This condition, and supposedly the etiology, is similar to Osgood-Schlatter's disease of the tibial tubercle. It also usually is noted in adolescent boys, with insidious onset of pain, tenderness, and some swelling over the inferior pole of the patella. The condition is aggravated by exercise or any activity that places stress on the patellar

104

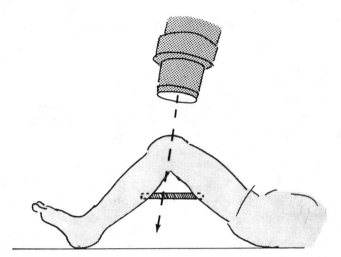

FIGURE 82. An x-ray skyline view for visualizing the femoral condyles.

tendon. In early stages, there are no bony changes noted on x-ray films but later an irregularity may be seen at the inferior pole.

Treatment consists of avoidance of activities by application of a cast if necessary. Usually six to eight weeks of inactivity eliminates the symptoms.

Osteochondritis Dissecans

This is a painful knee condition in which a fragment of articular cartilage with some subchondral bone separates partially or completely from the joint surface. The latter becomes a foreign body in the joint. It occurs in children, as an anomaly of ossification in adolescents (juvenile osteochondritis), or in adults. Men are most commonly affected.

Onset is usually insidious with pain described as aching and poorly localized; stiffness is claimed. When a loose body is present in the joint the knee can lock. Incidents of the knee giving way are frequent. This symptom is considered as an indication for surgical intervention.

Physical findings are sparse and nonspecific. There may be quadriceps atrophy, deep tenderness over the femoral condyle, and occasionally the loose body can be palpated. Diagnosis is verified by carefully x-raying the knee, with the use of tomograms if necessary.

Etiologic factors are:

1. Trauma from contact of the tibial tuberosity while striking the inner aspect of the femoral condyle or from a torn cartilage that narrows the joint.

105

2. Circulatory obstruction from thrombus or embolus (most unlikely as the condition frequently is bilateral).
3. Endocrine imbalance.
4. Heredity.

Differentiation of anomaly of ossification (age 10), juvenile osteochondritis (age 15), and osteochondritis dissecans (adult) aids the choice of treatment because time, rest, and immobilization cure the ossification anomaly but not always the other two.

X-ray films are diagnostic in that they indicate the presence of the condition and the site. Special views, such as the so-called tunnel view, are frequently needed. The various types and sites are shown in Figures 81 and 82.

Treatment in very young children consists of immobilization with a cylindrical cast, followed by serial x-ray studies. Surgical intervention consists of excision of the fragment, removal of the foreign body, or nailing of the fragment.

BIBLIOGRAPHY

AICHROTH, P: *Osteochondritis dissecans of the knee.* J Bone Joint Surg 53-B:440, 1971.

BENTLEY, G.: *Chondromalacia patellae.* J Bone Joint Surg 52-A:221, 1970.

BETZ, RR ET AL: The percutaneous lateral retinacular release. Orthopedics 5(1):57, 1982.

BLATZ, DJ, FLEMING, R, AND MCCARROLL, J: *Suprapatellar plica: A study of their occurrence and role in internal derangement of the knee in active duty personnel.* Orthopedics 4(2):181, February 1981.

CAVE, EF AND ROWE, CR: *The patella: Its importance in derangement of the knee.* J Bone Joint Surg 32-A:542, 1950.

CROOKS, LM: *Chondromalacia patellae: Early results of a conservative operation.* J Bone Joint Surg 49-B:495, 1967.

CROSBY, EB AND INSALL, J: *Recurrent dislocation of the patella. Relation of treatment to osteoarthritis.* J Bone Joint Surg 58-A(1):9, 1976.

DARRACOTT, J AND VERNON-ROBERTS, B: *The bony changes in "chondromalacia patellae."* Rheumatol Phys Med 11:175, 1971.

DATEL, D: *Arthroscopy of the plicae—synovial folds and their significance.* Am J Sports Med 6(5):217, 1978.

HILL, JA AND COMPERE, CL: *Comparative study of patellectomy.* Orthopedic Review. Vol X, No 3, 41-45, March 1981.

HOLLINGHEAD, WH: *Functional Anatomy of the Limbs and Back,* ed 2. WB Saunders, Philadelphia, 1960.

INSALL, J: *Curren Concepts Review Patellar Pain.* J Bone Joint Surg 64-A(1):147, 1982.

KAUFER, H: *Mechanical function of the patella.* J Bone Joint Surg 53-A, 1551, 1971.

MERCHANT, AC: *Isolated patellofemoral arthritis: Its significance and treatment.* Contemporary Orthopaedics 3(11):1015, 1981.

MISHRA, US: *Late results of patellectomy in fractured patella.* Acta Orthop Scand 43:256, 1972.

106

OSGOOD, RB: *Lesions of tibial tubercle occurring during adolescence.* Boston MSJ 148:114, 1903.

OUTERBRIDGE, RE: *Further studies on the etiology of chondromalacia patellae.* J Bone Joint Surg 46-B:179, 1964.

OUTERBRIDGE, RE: *The etiology of chondromalacia patellae.* J Bone Joint Surg 43-B:752, 1961.

PIPKIN, G: *Knee Injuries - The role of the suprapatellar plica and suprapatellar bursa in simulating internal derangements.* Clin Orthop 74:161, January 1971.

REILLY, DT AND MARTENS, M: *Experimental analysis of the quadriceps muscle force and patello-femoral joint reaction force for various activities.* Acta Orthop Scand 43:126, 1972.

SMILLIE, IS: *Osteochondritis dissecans of the knee.* Am J Orthop 6:236, 1964.

WIBERG, G: *Spontaneous healing of osteochondritis dissecans in the knee joint.* Acta Orthop Scand 14:270, 1943.

WIBERG, G: *Roentgenographic and anatomic studies on the patellofemoral joint with special reference to chondromalacia patellae.* Acta Orthop Scand 12:319, 1941.

WILPULLA, E AND VAHVANEN, V: *Chondromalacia of the patellae.* Acta Orthop Scand 42:521, 1971.

WORRELL, RV: *The diagnosis of disorders of the patellofemoral joint.* Orthopedic Review Vol X (3):73, 1981.

107

CHAPTER 6

Arthritides Affecting the Knee

RHEUMATOID ARTHRITIS

It is not the intent here to discuss arthritis in all its aspects: nomenclatures, classifications, etiologies, theories, and all their ramifications. These are the bases of large volumes and numerous articles and constitute the life studies of many authors. It is the purpose here to summarize that which is considered factual of the more prevalent types of arthritis, as they relate to the knee joint, for the purpose of diagnosis and better medical and surgical management.

Rheumatoid disease is a systemic disease: an inflammatory disorder of connective tissue with primary involvement of synovial membranes. Some organs of parenchymal tissue are involved as well as small arteries. Consideration here will be confined to the joints, tendons and their sheaths, and capsules (Fig. 83). The synovial tissues have limited ability to react and do so in a nonspecific manner. Rheumatoid disease does not elicit a specific pathognomic or diagnostic type of inflammation. The diagnosis of rheumatoid disease is thus possible on clinical ground with confirmation by laboratory tests. The criteria for diagnosis has been postulated by the American Rheumatism Association to include (1) morning stiffness, (2) pain on motion of joints, (3) symmetrical swelling of joints, (4) subcutaneous nodules, (5) typical changes seen on x-ray film, and (6) positive test for rheumatoid factor. Further revisions of these criteria are constantly under study.

Rheumatoid inflammation begins as congestion, edema, and cellular infiltration with plasma cella and lymphocytes predominating; in the acute phase, there may be a large proportion of polymorphs present. In the early phase of the disease, the joint surface may be covered with fibrinoid material while fibroblasts and capillaries invade the synovial tissue. This latter activity thickens the inflamed tissue and tends to organize the fibrinous tissue. The synovial fluid simultaneously undergoes in-

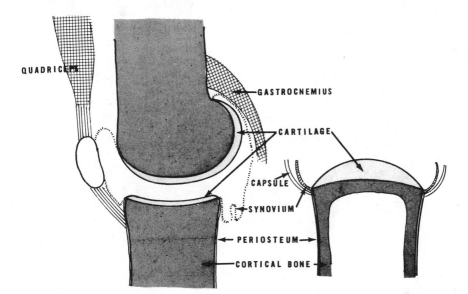

FIGURE 83. Knee joint structures: schematic. *Left,* Structures forming the joint; *Right,* Graphic illustration of the relationship of the capsule and the synovial membrane to the cartilaginous-cortical union.

flammatory reaction. The surrounding joint capsule and contiguous tendons and ligaments also undergo inflammatory reactions that, to this date being nonspecific, are considered to be physicochemical.

As the process continues, marginal erosions occur in the subchondral bone and the cartilage undergoes degenerative changes and pannus appears (Fig. 84).

Pannus is an apron of vascular granulation tissue consisting of proliferating fibroblasts, collagen fibers, small blood vessels, and numerous inflammatory cells. The current concept of articular damage and pannus formation is no longer considered to be cartilage destruction by the pannus but rather that cartilage destruction precedes pannus formation. Joints of acute rheumatoid arthritis of several weeks' duration have revealed articular matrix depletion and *no* pannus formation. There has even been expressed, the opinion that the pannus does not *invade* the cartilage but rather that it is formed from conversion of cartilage into fibrous tissue by metamorphosis of chondrocytes into fibroblasts. The exact mechanism of cartilage destruction is not known.

The interface between the pannus and the cartilage has been found to be crossed by fine collagen fibers, which may indicate that the pannus is not the destructive agent but rather is engaged in repairing the damaged cartilage with fibrous tissue. There are studies (Mills) that indicate that the granulation tissue that replaces the damaged cartilage is *not* a direct

109

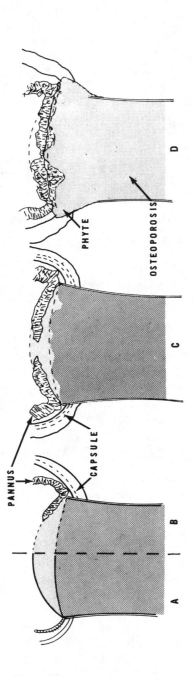

FIGURE 84. Progressive stages of rheumatoid disease of a joint. *A,* The normal half of a joint; *B,* Early thickening of the synovium, caused by edema, congestion, and invasion of fibroblasts and capillaries. The thickened synovium becomes termed pannus and gradually covers the cartilage. The capsule thickens. *C,* Pannus gradually invades and replaces the cartilage and the subchondral bone undergoes erosion. *D,* Advanced stage of the disease with loss of cartilage replaced by fibrous pannus, erosion of the subchondral bone, osteophyte (marginal) formation, and osteoporosis of the cortex. Only one bone that forms the joint has been shown, but the same condition is occurring in all the bones of the joint simultaneously.

extension of synovium but rather is invasion from the subchondral vascular spaces and from the marrow through the subchondral bone plate (Fig. 85). Pannus formation is considered to be a late phenomenon following the subchondral invasion. Synovial disease must initiate the process with all subsequent reactions being secondary.

Normally, the cartilage matrix consists of water, collagen, and protein polysaccharides. It is thought that the chondrocyte secretes the matrix, thus providing the rigidity and elasticity of the cartilage. The matrix is traversed by crisscrossing fibrils. The matrix has a limited life span and must be constantly renewed by the chondrocytes. Rheumatoid arthritis may arise from impairment of chondrocyte function as it furnishes the matrix (Fig. 86).

Lysosomes that contain enzymes capable of degrading all types of macromolecules (proteinases for proteins, carbohydrases, and lipases) are well surrounded by a membrane that holds in the enzymes. In rheumatoid disease, a *factor* is released that possibly ruptures the membrane and releases the enzymes that attack the chondrocytes. The factor possibly is chemical, an immunoglobulin, but presently is unknown. Rheumatoid disease also releases *fibrin,* a protein that may line the cartilage surface and deny entrance of the necessary nutrients.

Rheumatoid disease is currently considered to be an antigen-antibody reaction initiated by a bacterial or viral organism. It is this antigen-antibody reaction that releases the lysosome enzymes (see Fig. 86).

As the joint narrows from cartilage resorption the subchondral bone has and is undergoing erosion (see Fig. 84) with ultimate osteophyte formation at the margins. There is subsequent capsular thickening that combines with the fibrous replacement of the cartilage.

The ultimate stage of rheumatoid disease of the joint is either fibrous ankylosis or osteoarthritic degeneration with loss of all joint motion. The disease process may continue to ultimate destruction or stop at any stage, undergo some remission, have recurrences, or be aborted early before any destructive changes are evident.

History and Examination

The usual age of onset of rheumatoid arthritis is between 20 and 40 years, but there is a childhood form of the disease known as Still's disease, and onset has even been recorded in the sixth decade. The joints most frequently involved early in the disease are the hands and feet with the involvement being polyarticular and bilateral. In subsequent frequency of incidence come the wrists, ankles, elbows, and knees. Women are afflicted twice as often as men.

The disease is systemic. The patient appears ill, fatigues easily, and has poor appetite and poor nutrition. Anemia is prevalent. The patient is

111

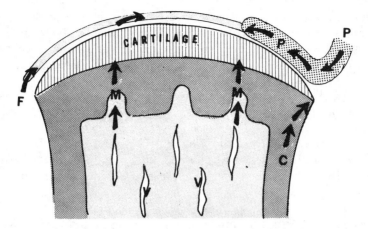

FIGURE 85. Schematic route of articular disease. The fibrinoid film *(F)* covers the cartilage and ultimately undergoes organization. Pannus *(P)*, which is inflamed synovium that contains fibroblasts and capillaries, has fine collagen fibers connecting to the cartilage. Marrow *(M)* and cortex *(C)* invasion of osteoclasts penetrate the subcortical bone plate to invade the cartilage and ultimately destroy it from within. *V* = deep blood vessels.

apprehensive and exhibits signs of vasomotor instability and poor muscle tone. The involved joints are swollen, warm, and tender and palpation reveals swelling with a periarticular bogginess. All joint motions (both active and passive) are avoided because of the pain that motion incites. Muscular atrophy is early and marked, as a manifestation of both the associated myopathic component of the disease and the disuse from pain, spasm, and ultimate articular contracture.

The onset systemically may be acute and fulminating or it may be insidious with slow gradual progression and occasional remission and recurrence. The type of disease progress cannot be predicted during the initial episode and no cause of exacerbation after a remission is known. The factors of fatigue, deconditioning, stress, and intercurrent infection have all been implicated.

Laboratory confirmation of the disease is made from elevation of the sedimentation rate: leukopenia (below 5000) is frequent but when there is leukocytosis there is predominance of lymphocytes. Hypoproteinemia occurs and the titer of rheumatoid factors is elevated.

Usually, the disease has been clinically evident and diagnosed before it is apparent that the knees are the principally involved joints. Synovial fluid drawn from the knee effusion is turbid with elevated specific gravity, slightly decreased sugar, and increase of cellular inclusion (usually polymorphs).

The disease follows a sequence of pathologic events (Fig. 87) in which all the tissues of and about the joint are involved simultaneously.

112

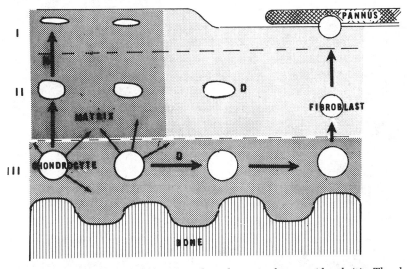

FIGURE 86. Schematic of theory of cartilage degradation in rheumatoid arthritis. The chondrocytes, located in the basal layers *(III)* secrete the matrix (primarily water, collagen, and protein polysaccharides). As the chondrocyte ages, it migrates *(arrows)* toward the joint space *(N)*. As degradation *(D)* occurs (cause unknown), the intermediate zone *(II)* loses metachromatic mucopolysaccharide (stains alkaline). A theory is expounded, which claims that some chondrocytes become fibroblasts that migrate peripherally to form the pannus. The pannus consists of vascular granulating tissue, proliferating fibroblasts, inflammatory cells, and collagen fibers. The chondrocytes may begin degradation when they are attacked by enzymes liberated from the lysosomes, which in turn were damaged by an infectious agent, for example, virus, bacteria.

Phase I: Soft tissue involvement. This is primarily synovial hyperemia with joint effusion. The surrounding ligaments and capsule are stretched, swollen, and tender. X-ray films taken at this stage merely reveal the soft tissue swelling with no articular changes.

Phase II: Continuation of synovitis, now with pannus formation and evidence of *nonarticular* bone destruction. It is at this stage that the synovium begins invasion of the cartilage and the adjacent bone. X-ray films here become diagnostic as there is noticeable bone destruction (erosion) at the margins of the articular cartilage under the collateral ligaments and appearance of decalcification. The joint space remains intact on routine x-ray study but arthroscopy would reveal the presence of pannus and some erosion of cartilage.

Phase III: Destruction of the cartilage and subchondral bone erosion. The joint space is now narrower; this is most apparent on the lateral aspect of the joint. Instability of the knee is now apparent. Soft tissue swelling has lessened because the synovial tissue is now more fibrotic and less

113

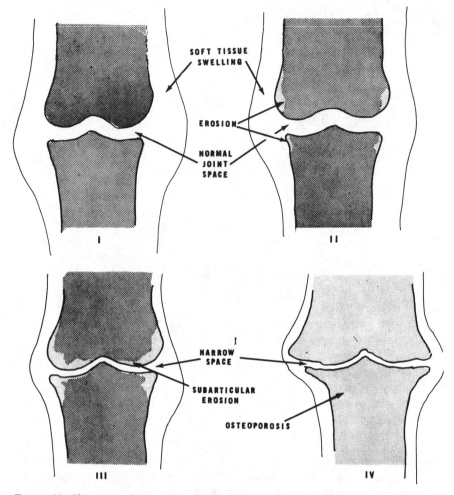

FIGURE 87. Changes in rheumatoid arthritis seen by x-ray study. *Phase I,* Early signs reveal soft tissue swelling with a normal joint space. Occasionally, the swelling may separate the involved joint. *Phase II,* As the disease progresses, some erosion is noted at the lateral margins where the collateral ligaments attach. *Phase III,* The erosion spreads centrally to the subchondral region, and the joint space narrows. *Phase IV,* The joint space becomes occluded as the cartilage completely disappears and bone opposes bone; the capsule is now fibrotic and not swollen (effused). There are bilateral osteophytes.

inflamed and vascular. The periarticular swelling is firmer and feels thicker.

Phase IV: Joint destruction of varying degree with marked cartilage destruction, which is apparent on x-ray film. There is marked joint laxity through ligamentous involvement which causes slackness as a result of the joint space narrowing.

Treatment

Treatment demands symptomatic medical treatment of rheumatoid disease; this will not be discussed in detail here. Suffice it to say that, in addition to a high protein diet, medication consists of salicylates, phenylbutazone, antimalarial drugs, gold salts, and steroids, dependent upon the experience of the treating physician. None as yet are specific. There are advocates of intra-articular injection of long-acting steroids. However, because this disease is prone to chronicity and recurrence and because repeated intra-articular steroids have been implicated in steroid arthropathy, the repeated use of steroids is not recommended as routine treatment.

Treatment of the knee afflicted with rheumatoid arthritis consists of physical methods with prevention of deformity as the goal. Unlike other joints that may be involved and for which complete *rest* of prolonged duration is valuable this tenet of complete rest and immobilization is not plausible in the knee. Flexion contraction, quadriceps atrophy, fibrous adhesions with possible ankylosis, and subluxation are frequent and severe; once established they are resistant to treatment. Reversibility of pathologic changes is difficult and often impossible.

EXERCISE. The position of flexion must be avoided during the acute phase. Unfortunately, this is the position of comfort to the patient; it is promoted by muscular spasm as well as joint capsular inflammation. Pillows must not be permitted under the knee during bedrest. Posterior mold splints can be made both to protect the extended knee and to afford comfort. The leg must be exercised periodically while in the splints. This can be done by assisted removal of the leg from the splint and gentle active and passive flexing and extending of the knee several times daily. This routine prevents intra-articular fibrosis and capsular contracture. Heat or ice applications as tolerated by the patient should accompany this daily ritual.

The quadriceps must be exercised immediately and frequently and with effort in this disease. The type of exercise best tolerated in the *acute* joint phase is that of quadriceps setting (isometric) straight-leg raising within the cast and during the period when the cast is removed. A gradual increase of this quadriceps activity to active isotonic resisted exercises should be made as tolerated. Weight bearing should be avoided except with the aid of crutches or walker and should be strictly avoided if any flexion contracture exists. Use of braces or cages, which immobilize the extended knee, is to be discouraged because it adds to further atrophy and dependence.

Upon subsidence or decrease of inflammation with its resultant spasm and painful joint motion, active exercises should be instituted. These are similar to the exercises described in Chapter 3. Once resistive exercises are initiated they should be carefully supervised, done frequently during the

115

day, and gradually *increased with encouragement*. Patient fear and low threshold of pain are strong factors that delay progress in rehabilitation efforts. Fear that pain means aggravation of the disease must be allayed and constant encouragement should be given. After remission or subsidence of the acute phase of the illness, a progressive exercise program must be maintained in order to minimize any possible exacerbation that, being superimposed on a partial residual disability, could have detrimental disabling effects.

ASPIRATION. During the acute stages of phases I or II, significant effusion should be aspirated because its persistence will overdistend the capsule and ligaments and limit range of joint motion. Passive and active exercises during effusion are limited.

The technique of intra-articular aspiration is relatively simple but justifies clarification. Aseptic conditions are mandatory because an arthritic joint with superimposed infection can be calamitous. Entrance preferably is made from the lateral side. The patella is passively moved toward the lateral side, which widens the joint space between the patella and the femoral condyle (Fig. 88).

Normally, there is insufficient synovial fluid to aspirate. In effusion or hemarthrosis the leg can be placed with the lateral margin down. This can be accomplished by laterally rotating the reclining patient. Gravity causes the fluid to seek a dependent position. An 18-gauge needle is inserted into the suprapatellar pouch. By also injecting air (approximately 10 ml) and then applying manual pressure in the popliteal space, the fluid is further brought to the needle. The needle can be withdrawn slowly while aspirating to completely evacuate the fluid.

The initial tapped fluid should be studied for cell count, presence of crystals, sugar, mucin, and other pertinent diagnostic studies. Intra-articular steroids at the time of aspiration is questionable because the benefit is not fully accepted and the detrimental effect of intra-articular steroids, especially if repeated, is well documented.

SURGERY. Findings that indicate continued active synovitis and persistence of symptoms *after six months* (arbitrarily determined) indicate the desirability of synovectomy. The efficacy of synovectomy has not been proven in halting the systemic ravages of the disease nor in preventing recurrences. However, it is an accepted fact that synovectomy does delay damage to the articular cartilage, may initiate a remission of the disease, and possibly decreases the synovial reaction of other joints simultaneously affected. Synovectomy does *not* damage an intact joint and it does prevent phase I of the rheumatoid joint from advancing into phases II and III.

Synovectomy in phase III probably does not decrease further degenerative changes but does aid in joint management when performed also for the sake of debridement. In phase III careful consideration must be given

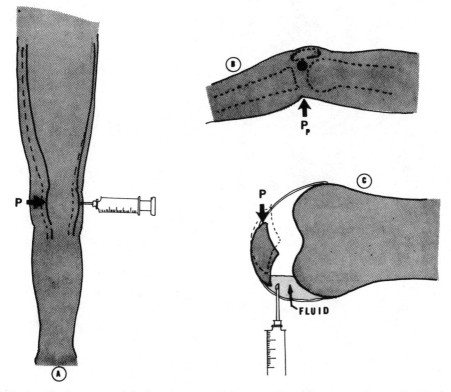

FIGURE 88. Aspiration of the knee joint. A, Technique of laterally moving the patella (P) to increase the injectable space between the patella and the femoral condyle. B, Lateral view, site of injection (black dot) and popliteal space pressure (P_p) to bring fluid to needle tip. C, With lateral position, the fluid gravitates to permit easier aspiration.

regarding arthroplasty prosthesis. At this date, the devices used are the McIntosh or McKeever prostheses or the femoral condyle prosthesis of Aufranc. Total knee replacements have not been proven in the number done and duration of their use to be recommended.

The aim of arthroplasty is to alleviate pain, correct deformity, and increase joint range of motion. Hemiarthrodesis aims to correct a varus or valgus deformity (Fig. 89). A tibial plateau prosthesis of proper width realigns the joint, creates a smooth painless gliding surface and adheres to the tibia by virtue of its serrated undersurface. When the joint is physiologically realigned, the ligaments resume their normal length. The collateral ligaments do not lose their normal length in long-standing varus or valgus deformity. Prosthesis should be considered *only* when synovectomy, debridement, or tibial osteotomy have been considered and found of no value or when there is no remaining cartilage and bone is rubbing against bone. The prosthesis becomes covered with a layer of fibrous tissue that

117

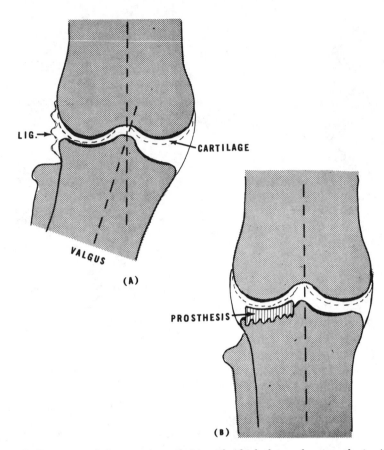

FIGURE 89. Treatment of degenerative arthritis with tibial plateau hemiprosthesis. A, The usual valgus of the degnerated knee joint with marked narrowing of the lateral joint compartment. The capsule is redundant. B, Insert of the prosthesis straightens the knee and separates the lateral joint space.

forms an envelope around it and helps bind it down. Postoperative success may depend on this development.

Prostheses are contraindicated when there has been a previous plateau fracture or previous infection or fusion, when a neurotrophic arthritis exists, or when there is questionable patient cooperation. Severe joint destruction may be a contraindication; arthroscopy here may help verify the existence of remaining cartilage.

Arthrodesis will provide a stable and pain-free knee; it is a salvage operation that is considered the final solution. However, recommendation of this procedure depends on the condition of the other joint of the extremity and the ability of the patient to function adequately with the other knee. Preoperatively, the involved knee can be temporarily immobilized by casting as a test of the patient's functional ability and acceptance of the inability to flex the knee. Further involvement of the remaining uninvolved knee may cause irreversible disability and precludes other surgery short of total knee replacement.

OSTEOARTHRITIS (DEGENERATIVE ARTHRITIS), OSTEOARTHROSIS

Osteoarthritis, also commonly called degenerative arthritis or osteoarthrosis, connotes joint disease that is degenerative as compared to inflammatory or infectious. It is thus differentiated from rheumatoid arthritis and its variants. Osteoarthritis is differentiated as primary (idiopathic) or secondary to a preceding infectious, traumatic, inflammatory, metabolic, or aging process. Regardless of classification, the pathomechanics of the joint disease are not known.

Osteoarthritis is essentially a degenerative condition of the joint articular cartilage with subsequent formation of marginal osteophytes, subchondral bone changes, bone marrow changes, fibrous reaction of the synovium, and capsular thickening.

Early degenerative changes may be asymptomatic until synovitis develops with effusion, stiffness, capsular thickening, and formation of marginal osteophytes. Pain is considered to be caused by the stretching of the periosteum by the expanding osteophytes, bony changes at points of ligamentous attachment, and the protective muscle spasm that occurs to immobilize the painful joint.

Certain changes occur in aging of articular cartilage that are difficult to differentiate from osteoarthritic changes. These changes differ from person to person, joint to joint, and from various areas of the opposing articular surfaces. There are generalized changes in the joint destructive process as well as focal cartilage changes. Normal joints undergo *maturation* that defies differentiation from degenerative changes. Joints are constantly undergoing normal remodeling, a process of wear and repair, which is considered to be a destructive process when an imbalance occurs between destruction and repair.

Of the many concepts considered to be causative factors in osteoarthritis, the most attractive and acceptable is that which postulates that synovitis represents chronic chemical inflammation of the cartilage resulting from excessive concentration of polysaccharides formed in the joint from debris of damaged cartilage (Fig. 90). This theory has been reproduced experimentally by injecting debris of scraped cartilage intra-articularly with resultant synovitis, capsular thickening, loss of cartilage elasticity (because of loss of protein polysaccharides), fissuring, and ultimate fibrillation with gradual denuding of the cartilage to the depths of subchondral bone.

119

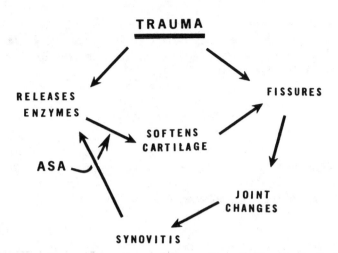

FIGURE 90. Schematic process in progress of degenerative arthritis: site of salicylate action.

Fibrillation occurs from vertical fissures that penetrate toward sub-chondral bone. A loss of mucopolysaccharides may precede or follow the fissuring. The subchondral bone becomes hyperemic and blood vessels containing fibrous tissue penetrate the subchondral plate and enter the denuding cartilage. The idea that metachromatic mucopolysaccharide loss is greatest in the midtransitional zone of the cartilage implies enzymic penetration rather than surface friction as the cause of wear and tear. A proteolytic (collagenase) enzyme appears to be the causative factor.

Salicylates act as an enzyme inhibitor that prevents chondromalacia. This has been documented both clinically and experimentally and when given early and in adequate doses prevents fibrillation. Once fibrillation is established, salicylates are ineffective. This fact and other studies indicate that chemical as well as mechanical factors play a major part in osteoarthritis.

Treatment of degenerative arthritis is not complicated but requires attention to details. Mere control of the inflammatory state may leave an unstable knee joint. Heat application is usually beneficial in this type of arthritis and may be applied by hot moist packs, diathermy, or a baker. Weight reduction is mandatory. Evaluation of the patient's daily activities must be thoroughly studied and necessary changes made. Low chairs must be avoided and the patient must not remain in the same position for prolonged periods of time. Upon awakening in the morning, active flexion and extension of the knee should be done before weight bearing is attempted.

Walking should be encouraged for daily activities but not forced for the sake of prolonged exercise as a therapy. Deep knee bends also should be avoided. Faulty posture that places a strain on the stance should be cor-

120

rected. Exercises should be a daily ritual to strengthen the quadriceps extensor group by setting exercises increasing to full progressive resistive exercises as tolerated. Hamstring exercises with the patient standing, holding on to a dresser or table, and flexing the knee 20 times or to the point of fatigue are beneficial. In the same position gastrocnemius-soleus exercises are performed, in which the patient rises on the toes of both feet simultaneously, one foot alternately, and progresses to toe raising from a book placed under the ball of the foot.

If the patient has a severe valgus or varus of the knee with severe narrowing of the joint on the concave side, osteotomy of the tibia and fibula can relieve the patient's symptoms by shifting weight to the opposite side of the joint.

HEMOPHILIC ARTHRITIS

Hemophilia is an abnormal hemorrhaging condition with hereditary and familial tendencies sustained by men and transmitted by women. Essentially, the disease is a failure of blood to clot with a resultant period of excessive bleeding. Hemarthrosis, bleeding into the joint, is common and presents a major adversity of the disease with resultant disability.

Onset of hemophilia is usually between ages 4 to 10 and is noted initially as a sequela of trauma. The knee, because of its exposure to stress and injury, frequently is involved and hemarthrosis of the knee is often the first evidence of the disease.

Acute hemarthrosis manifests itself by a rapid swelling of the joint, intense pain, and marked muscle spasm. The joint capsule becomes markedly distended with concomitant swelling of the periarticular tissues. The knee is hot and extremely sensitive and rapidly demonstrates a tight, taut skin over the entire joint. Hemorrhage may become so severe as to rupture through the capsule and penetrate the periarticular soft tissue with ecchymosis and even tissue sloughing.

Intra-articular hemorrhage invades all the intra-articular tissues. Besides damage resulting from the intense distension from the blood, the blood elements irritate the synovial membrane from a toxic effect not fully understood. Blood pigments impregnate the synovium, which changes color, texture, and thickness. The synovium may undergo hyperplasia with formation of villi. Usually, the first bout(s) of hemarthrosis subsides and the synovium returns to its normal state. With repeated episodes, the synovium is invaded by fibrous elements, undergoes hypertrophy, and thickens into a hyperplastic tissue.

Repeated hemarthrosis ultimately affects the cartilage adversely, possibly by (1) damage as a result of excessive unremittent pressure of the increased synovial fluid, (2) impairment of the nutritive aspect of the

121

synovial fluid, and (3) toxic elements considered to exist in hemophiliac blood. The latter possibility has not been confirmed.

The cartilage thins and ultimately erodes to the subchondral bone (Fig. 91), causing subchondral sclerosis and cysts. These cysts are considered to be hemorrhaging into the bone cortex. They are noted on x-ray films and are especially prominent in the region of the tibial plateau.

In chronic cases, the entire joint may become obliterated by firm fibrous adhesions extending from the tibial to the femoral condyles. This thick pannus is fibrous tissue that grows from the subchondral bone through the crevices in the cartilage. Fibrous ankylosis may be the inevitable result.

Flexion deformity occurs early in the affected extremity. The distended capsule and the concomitant hamstring spasm tend to flex the knee, which gives some relief of pain to the patient but on the other hand enhances further disability. With recurrent episodes of hemarthrosis, the posterior capsule thickens and thus maintains flexion deformity. Ambulation in this flexed knee position places abnormal stress upon the articular tissues and adds to the deformity.

Treatment of hemophilic arthritis of the knee includes treatment of hemophilia as well as care for other hemorrhagic sites that may have more drastic residual. Immediate administration of plasma products is imperative following diagnosis. These products must be available. A center for treatment of hemophiliacs may exist in the community; its presence should be known. The products currently recommended: for hemophilia A, AHF plasma concentrate or AHF cryoprecipitate; for hemophilia B (PTC or Factor IX deficiency), plasma concentrate if available. Plasma may be used but it is difficult to elevate the AHF level to sufficient hemostatic level with its use. The dosage of plasma products is based on severity of bleeding and patient's weight, thus insuring a minimum of 30 percent AHF to PTC level. Care and good technique in administration are mandatory.

Care of the knee itself is a tedious procedure. Many aspects of treatment may seem feasible yet be instrumental in causing more bleeding. Enforced rest of the knee is mandatory with elevation, cold compresses (possibly ice), and gentle but firm and uniform compression bandaging.

Aspiration of the hemorrhaging articular fluid as an isolated procedure may increase bleeding and therefore must be done after administration of plasma concentrates that raise the level of AHF to 50 percent. It must be done with extreme care of asepsis. Intra-articular instillation of steroid or hyaluronidase has proven to be effective in enhancing absorption of the hemarthrosis, relieving pain simultaneously, and permitting earlier gradual motion. Its instillation into the joint also minimizes the proliferative changes in the synovium, which are the precursor of ultimate fibrosis. The mode of action of hyaluronidase is not fully understood but it appar-

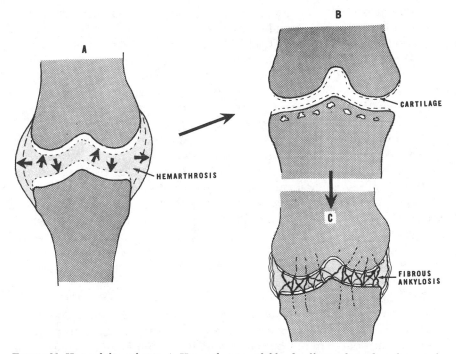

FIGURE 91. Hemophilic arthritis. *A*, Hemarthrosis with bloody effusion distending the capsule and putting pressure *(arrows)* against the cartilage of the femur and the tibia. *B*, If there is persistence or frequent recurrence of hemarthrosis, the cartilage thins. *C*, Chronic stage with fibrous reaction within the bloody effusion, organization of the hemorrhagic effusion, fibrous invasion through the damaged cartilage, and ultimate fibrous ankylosis.

ently enhances interchange of articular fluid through its effect upon the mucopolysaccharide of the cartilage. It also decreases the viscosity of the synovial fluid and possibly through these and other actions increases the permeability of the synovial membrane.

Hyaluronidase instillation must be aseptically performed. An equal amount of hyaluronidase mixed with 1 percent procaine (or derivative) is added to 4 to 6 ml of the aspirated fluid and is injected into the joint through the same needle. No further fluid is aspirated. Following the instillation, a firm elastic bandage, which exerts uniform, firm but gentle pressure, is applied and the joint is rested in an elevated position for 24 hours. Persistence of pain and spasm is an indication for a repeat aspiration and instillation in 24 hours.

Pain and swelling usually diminish within 24 hours of the first instillation. In this case, a gentle active and passive range of joint motion is encouraged and closely supervised. When the joint is moved frequently with gradual increase of extent, there is diminution of fibrosis, capsular

123

thickening, and ultimate ankylosis. Other parenteral and oral antihemor-rhagic medications are administered.

With levels of AHF or PTC of 50 percent at the time of aspiration, this procedure can be performed on an outpatient basis. A second dose of plasma concentrate must be given on the fourth or fifth day post-aspiration to assure a level of 20 to 30 percent. Twenty-four hours of joint immobilization must be maintained after the aspiration. Some support to the knee may be required for ambulation during the first 24 hours.

Even though elective corrective surgery may now be performed where plasma concentrates are available, the intent is toward prevention of deformity. During the acute phase of hemorrhage, the knee can be splinted with a carefully applied well-padded splint with a flexible wire to maintain and increase the range of extension (Fig. 92). The splint may be adjusted daily. A posterior mold splint is effective but must be remade frequently to adjust to the desired angle. Active exercises should be started to maintain or increase quadriceps strength as soon as swelling and pain have subsided. These exercises can be isometric initially with gradual increase to isotonic and resisted.

Retroperitoneal hemorrhage is frequent and may occur in the iliopsoas area, causing femoral nerve damage and hypaesthesia and quadriceps paresis. This should be suspected when there is severe quadriceps weakness and atrophy. Plasma products must be continued to maintain levels of AHF for at least 7 to 10 days. Traction to the hip should *not* be instituted as it may increase bleeding. Quadriceps exercises should be started shortly, preferably in a pool area. Weight bearing should be avoided until hip flexion is less than 25°. If quadriceps paralysis is severe some support may be needed when ambulation is begun.

After fibrous ankylosis to the knee is apparent an active exercise and corrective bracing program (see Fig. 92) usually results in gratifying improvement. If ankylosis is severe and fails to improve, it is generally considered desirable to allow natural ankylosis to occur in the most physiologic position rather than attempt surgical arthrodesis.

GOUTY ARTHRITIS

Gout is a hereditary metabolic disease predominantly afflicting men, carried and transmitted by women. Clinically, the disease becomes apparent in adult life between ages 35 to 50. Many relatives of patients with gout have hyperuricemia but never develop clinical manifestations.

Uric acid is known to be a threshold substance formed by the body, eliminated by the renal glomeruli, circulated in the blood, and reabsorbed partly by the kidney tubules. There are three postulated internal dysfunctions that lead to increased uric acid concentration in tissue fluids:

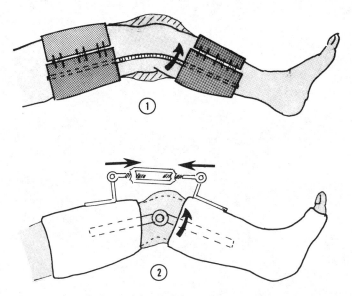

FIGURE 92. Corrective splinting of hemophilic arthritis. *1*, During the acute phase of hemarthrosis, a splint, consisting of a thigh and a lower leg thermoplastic shell held by Velcro straps, can be connected with a flexible wire that can be bent to gradually extend the knee. The knee is visible and change can be made immediately upon an increase of hemorrhage. *2*, A plaster cast, hinged at the knee, can be made for chronic fibrous contracture of the knee in varying degrees of flexion. Gradual extension is obtained by a dorsal turnbuckle that can be turned gradually several times a day or a few degrees every other day as tolerated.

1. Diminished excretion by the kidneys: decreased glomerular filtration or increased reabsorption by the tubules.
2. Excessive formation of urates as a result of faulty metabolism.
3. Diminished destruction of urates by faulty enzymes.

An excess of urates in the serum does not constitute gout until these urates are deposited into mesenchymal tissues through a chemical or metabolic mechanism. Why and how this alteration of urates occurs is not known. An electrolyte imbalance converting uric acid to a sodium urate is postulated: monosodium urate [Na $(C_5H_3O_3N_4) \bullet H_2O$].

Urate crystal deposits are prone to develop in avascular rather than vascular tissues, thus its predilection for cartilage, bursae, ligaments, tendons, and epiphysial portions of bone. Tophi (accumulations of urates) are conspicuously absent from muscle, lungs, liver, nervous tissue, and kidneys. Urate crystals are deposited in the superficial layers of the cartilage, causing fibrillation. The cartilage *overlying* the deposit is destroyed (Fig. 93) releasing the crystals into the joint space and into the synovial fluid.

125

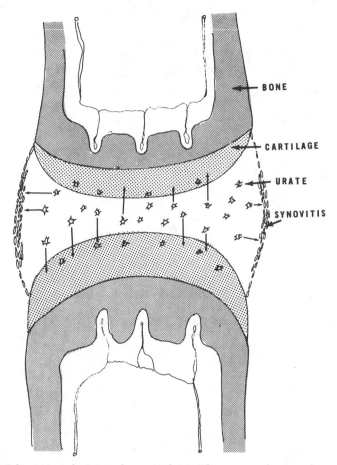

BONE

CARTILAGE

URATE

SYNOVITIS

FIGURE 93. Schematic explanation of gouty arthritis. The exact mechanism of gouty arthritis is not verified. The currently accepted theory is that urate crystals form in the synovial fluid and penetrate the outer layer of the cartilage, depositing crystals there. Urate crystals also irritate the synovial layer, causing synovitis. Migration of urates via the subchondral epiphyseal bone is not currently accepted.

While still within the superficial layers of the cartilage, the tophus becomes surrounded by granulation tissue, leukocytes, round cells, and giant cells. There is also surrounding edema and hyperemia. This inflammation and its subsequent emission into the joint fluid softens the tophus. Less than 50 percent of patients with gout exhibit tophi.

During the acute attack, a thin pannus forms from the synovium covering the cartilage surface. There is an increase in synovial fluid and concomitant periarticular inflammation. Clinically, the joint is swollen, reddened, and tense with overlying taut, shiny skin. Attack is usually sudden with severely painful swelling and discoloration. Involvement is characteristically in *one* joint, a fact that is of diagnostic significance in differentiating the acute onset of rheumatoid arthritis. The latter is multiarticular and bilateral with symmetrical involvement and usually is found in women or in emaciated sick patients. The acute attack of gout usually subsides within four to seven days leaving a normal joint upon subsidence of the inflammation. Repeated attacks leave permanent damage with joint changes similar to those noted in osteoarthritis.

Attacks have been considered as resulting from trauma, overexertion, dietary or alcoholic excesses, surgical procedures elsewhere in the body, or after severe diuresis (usually from use of mercurial salt diuretics).

X-ray studies are not pathognomonic. They reveal similar changes noted in early rheumatoid or degenerative arthritis, but when cysts are noted near the articular margins they are probably masses of urate crystals.

The diagnosis of gouty arthritis consists of a typical history of an acute, *mono*articular, swollen joint with systemic symptoms of fever and leukocytosis. Occurrence is in men of 35 to 50 years of age in otherwise good health. Uric acid in the serum usually is elevated and crystals may be found in the aspirated joint fluid.

Treatment is prophylactic in regards to systemic treatment. It includes dietary restrictions to avoid purine-rich foods and fats, avoidance of obesity, avoidance of diuretics, and oral administration of colchicine, benemid, or both. During the acute episode these drugs, as well as butazolidin or steroids, may be used depending upon the experience of the treating physician.

Care of the involved knee joint is symptomatic. The knee must be immobilized. Effusion, if marked, should be aspirated. A posterior mold splint and cold compresses are effective. Compression dressings usually are poorly tolerated. Recovery after the acute episode is usual with no residual.

PYOGENIC ARTHRITIS

Suppurative arthritis is usually secondary to septicemia or secondary to local invasion. The organism may be identified by joint fluid examination, culture, or blood culture. Treatment demands proper and specific antibiotic administration. Infection into the joint from adjacent bone or soft tissue involvement must be approached by care of that focal point.

The purulent joint must be aspirated (repeatedly if necessary) and antibiotics instilled into the joint as well as given orally or parenterally. The joint must be rested but *flexion must be avoided.* A posterior molded splint may be effective coupled with hot fomentations. Traction is useful to immobilize the knee, maintain adequate extension, and maintain joint surface distraction. As soon as inflammation subsides and allows it, exer-

127

cise for the quadriceps must be initiated. Ultimately, rehabilitation, as in all arthritides, must be considered.

NEOPLASMS ABOUT THE KNEE

Both primary and metastatic lesions must be considered when pain, deformity, and disability occur in or around the knee joint. Numerous classifications of neoplasms are available in current literature. Diagnosis is made by careful history, taking meticulous examination, x-ray study repeated as often as necessary, isotope scan studies, biopsy, blood chemistry studies, and search for primary lesion. Treatment is eventually *the* considered specific treatment for that neoplastic type, extent, duration, and other oncologic aspects of the disease.

BURSITIS

Any of the bursae (described in Chapter 1) can become inflamed, swollen, and cause symptoms. Any of these bursae can be swollen and symptomatic or merely noted in the course of routine examination as an asymptomatic swelling. Several types of acute, chronic, or recurrent bursitis about the knee warrant discussion.

The prepatellar bursa lies between the skin and the outer surface of the patella and is prone to direct trauma from a fall or kneeling. Diagnosis from these causes is usually easy with local tenderness, swelling, and inflammation as symptoms. Pain is usually present from tension of the skin in extreme knee flexion or by direct pressure. Treatment for this type of bursitis is usually conservative, it occasionally requires aspiration but rarely does it need incision and drainage. Chronic prepatellar bursitis that results from repeated bouts of irritation may be more recalcitrant to conservative treatment. Drainage followed by pressure dressing and protective padding may be effective. Occasionally, total excision of the inflamed thickened bursa is necessary.

Deep infrapatellar bursitis usually occurs from overactivity with undue friction against the upper tibia. This deep bursitis rarely results from direct trauma as the bursa is well protected by the overlying patella and the underlying fat pad. Tenderness can be elicited by pressure *behind* the infrapatellar tendon and from passive forced flexion and active extension of the knee. Treatment is supportive and consists of heat, immobilization, and aspiration. Occasionally, instillation of steroids is used but its efficacy is equivocal. Excision is considered when conservative treatment fails.

All other sites of bursitis about the knee usually can be diagnosed by appropriate examination and localizing signs *if bursitis is suspected.*

Posterior bursitis occurs when there are cystic tumors of the popliteal space. The tumors have been termed popliteal or synovial cysts, posterior bursae, Baker's cysts, or semimembranous or gastrocnemius-membrano-sus bursae. Various authors have claimed from 7 to 50 percent of normal population show communication between the joint space and this posterior popliteal bursa during arthrography. These cysts may include bursal effusion between the medial head of the gastrocnemius and the semimembranosus tendon, which may in turn communicate with the capsule space.

The cause of these popliteal cysts is probably that of normal anatomic connection aggravated by chronic effusion of the intra-articular joint cavity. Chronic effusion may be caused by rheumatoid arthritis, meniscus tear, cruciate ligamentous tears, and so forth. The incidence of these cysts increase with aging but there is no significant sexual difference.

Treatment of this cyst consists of treatment of the underlying cause. Investigation by arthrography or arthrotomy of any internal articular disease or damage must precede any treatment directed to the cyst. Originally, treatment was comprised of excision of the cyst with closure of the communication; this no longer is considered valid in the common cyst. However, if the cyst is large and causing inconvenience it can be aspirated and compressed or it can be totally excised.

BIBLIOGRAPHY

BIGGS, R AND MACFARLANE, RG: *Treatment of Hemophila and Other Coagulation Disorders.* FA Davis, Philadelphia, 1966.

BRATTSTROM, M: *Asymmetry of ossification and rate of growth of long bones in children with unilateral juvenile gonarthritis.* Acta Rheum Scand 9:102, 1963.

BYER, PD: *The pathology of rheumatic diseases.* In LIGHT, S (ED): *Arthritis and Physical Medicine.* Licht, New Haven, 1969, Ch 3.

CAMPBELL, CJ: *The healing of cartilage defects.* Clin Orthop 64:45, 1969.

CHRISMAN, OD: *Biochemical aspects of degenerative joint disease.* Clin Orthop 64:77, 1969.

CONVERY, FR: *The rheumatoid knee.* Am Fam Physician 4:52, 1971.

COVENTRY, MB: *Osteotomy about the knee for degenerative and rheumatoid arthritis.* J Bone Joint Surg 55-A(1):23, 1973.

ENNEKING, WF AND HOROWITZ, M: *The intra-articular effects of immobilization on the human knee.* J Bone Joint Surg 54-A:973, 1972.

EYRING, EJ: *The therapeutic potential of synovectomy in juvenile rheumatoid arthritis.* Arthritis Rheum 11:688, 1968.

GHORMLEY, RK AND CLEGG, RS: *Bone and joint changes in hemophila.* J Bone Joint Surg 30-A:589, 1948.

GOLDIE, I AND SCHLOSSMAN, D: *Radiological changes in rheumatoid knee joints before and after synovectomy.* Clin Orthop 64:98, 1969.

HALL, MC: *Cartilaginous changes after experimental relief of contact in the knee joint of the mature rat.* Clin Orthop 64:64, 1969.

JACKSON, RW AND ABE, I: *The role of arthroscopy in management of disorders of the knee.* J Bone Joint Surg 54-B:310, 1972.

KAY, NRM AND MARTINS, HD: *The MacIntosh tibial plateau hemiprosthesis for the rheumatoid knee.* J Bone Joint Surg 54-B:256, 1972.

MACINTOSH, DL AND HUNTER, GA: *The use of the hemiarthroplasty prosthesis for advanced osteoarthritis and rheumatoid arthritis of the knee.* J Bone Joint Surg 54-B:244, 1972.

MARMOR, L: *Osteoarthritis of the knee.* JAMA 318:213, 1971.

MARMOR, L: *Surgery of Rheumatoid Arthritis.* Henry Kimpton, London, 1967.

MARSHALL, JL AND OLSON, CE: *Instability of the knee: A long term experimental study in dogs.* J Bone Joint Surg 53-A:1561, 1971.

MCCARTY, DJ, HOGAN, JN, GATTEN, R AND GROSSMAN, M: *Studies on pathological calcifications in human cartilage.* J Bone Joint Surg 48-A:309, 1966.

MCKEEVER, DC: *Tibial plateau prosthesis.* Clin Orthop 18:86, 1960.

MCMASTER, M: *Synovectomy of the knee in juvenile rheumatoid arthritis.* J Bone Joint Surg 54-B:262, 1972.

MILLS, K: *Pathology of the knee joint in rheumatoid arthritis.* J Bone Joint Surg 52-B:746, 1970.

SHANDS, AR: *Neuropathies of the bones and joints.* Arch Surg 20:614, 1930.

SHERMAN, MS: *The non-specificity of synovial reactions.* Bull Hosp Joint Dis 12:110, 1951.

SMITH, CF et al: *Long-term management and rehabilitation in hemophilia. Project report, PH Grant 110-91.* Orthopedic Hospital, Los Angeles, 1969.

WILSON, PD, EYRE-BROOK, AL, AND FRANCIS, JD: *A clinical and anatomical study of the semimembranosus bursa in relation to popliteal cyst.* J Bone Joint Surg 20:963, 1938.

WOLFE, RD AND COLLOFF, B: *Popliteal cysts, an arthrographic study and review of the literature.* J Bone Joint Surg 54-A(5):1057, 1972.

CHAPTER 7

Fractures About the Knee Joint

No treatise of the knee would be complete without discussion of fractures about the knee joint. Some of these fractures may be very complicated and present difficulties in their management, thus full dissertation of all these aspects cannot be covered in this brief chapter. Only basic types and basic principles of their management will be undertaken.

Fractures about the knee may be classified in various categories regarding fractures of the distal end of the femur, proximal end of the tibia, and the patella. Fractures of the distal end of the femur may be divided into supracondylar, intercondylar, and condylar (Fig. 94). Fractures of the tibial plateau may be divided into those (1) involving the lateral condyle or the medial condyle, (2) with or without comminution or displacement, and (3) with variable degrees of depression.

Fractures about the knee must also be evaluated in respect to the injury sustained by the cartilage: chondral fractures involving only the articular cartilage or osteochondral fractures involving the articular cartilage and the underlying subchondral bone. Sudden violent stress can cause avulsion fracture in which a fragment of bone is avulsed by its attachment to a tendon or ligament.

Etiologic factors of fractures can be torsion injuries with the fixed foot internally or externally rotated in relationship to the femur, caused by direct violence, or cartilage damage secondary to subluxation of the patella.

Symptoms consist of effusion (hemarthrosis), pain, localized tenderness, crepitation, locking, and varying degrees of disability. X-ray films may be diagnostic but may be unrewarding in chondral fractures. Arthrography may show radiolucent filling defect when a fracture is suspected. Management obviously depends upon the exact mechanism of fracture, the alignment of the fragments, the articular integrity, and proper joint surface alignment. Basic principles must underly all treatment such as removal of fragment, removal of associated meniscus tear,

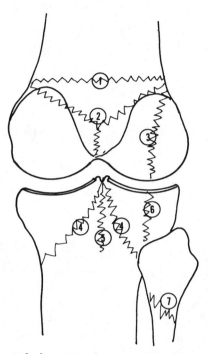

FIGURE 94. Fractures about the knee joint: fractures of distal femur and proximal tibia. *1*, Supracondylar fracture; *2*, Intercondylar fracture Y type; *3*, Condylar fracture of femur; *4*, Condylar fracture of tibial plateau; *5*, Intercondylar vertical fracture of tibial plateau; *6*, Condylar fracture of medial or lateral tibia; and *7*, Fibular fracture.

replacement of the fragment with internal fixation, and reconstruction of the extensor mechanism.

FRACTURES OF DISTAL END OF FEMUR

Anatomically, the distal end of the femur comprises two large rounded condyles covered with cartilage (see Chapter 1). Muscular attachment about the joint influences the resultant fracture fragments and their alignment. The gastrocnemius muscle pulls the distal fragment posteriorly (Fig. 95) toward the nerves and the blood vessels of the popliteal fossa. The collateral ligaments are frequently involved in the mechanism of fracture and must always be fully evaluated in determination of the extent of the fracture. Effusion (hemarthrosis) of the knee joint usually is present. Soft tissue must always be considered in prolonged immobilization with fragments in proper alignment because of the possibility of muscular atrophy (quadriceps femorus) and intra-articular adhesions. Improper realignment of the cartilage surface may lead to ultimate arthritic changes (a complication possible even with the best of alignment).

132

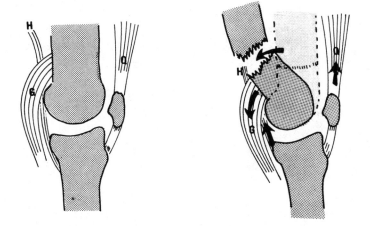

FIGURE 95. Muscular action upon fracture fragments: supracondylar fracture. *Left,* Muscular action about the knee joint. *Right,* Action of the gastrocnemius, pulling the distal fragment posteriorly into the popliteal fossa and the hamstring and quadriceps pulling longitudinally to shorten the femur.

G = Gastrocnemius
H = Hamstrings
Q = Quadriceps

Supracondylar Fractures

This type of fracture is usually caused by direct violence or torsion stress. Usually there is displacement of the fragments (see Fig. 95) caused by muscular action; the gastrocnemius pulling the distal fragment posteriorly into the fossa and the hamstrings and quadriceps shortening the length of the femur.

Management may be by closed reduction or open reduction, with the former usually possible and desirable. Alignment is attempted on a fracture table and with skeletal traction. If the joint is distended with blood, it is aspirated under sterile technique. The hip is flexed (45 to 60°) (Fig. 96). The flexed lower leg tends to reduce the posterior displacement and manual pressure completes this displacement. After reduction, a plaster spica is applied with the knee in the flexed position and the wires incorporated into the plaster. Wires are usually removed in four to six weeks and the cast removed in six to eight weeks.

In cases that defy reduction, continuous traction in a Bohler-Braun splint may be necessary. The principles are the same as those just discussed. The gained position of reduction can usually be maintained with 10 to 12 lb of traction but as much as 20 to 25 lb of traction for 24 to 48 hours may be necessary. Because muscular atrophy of the quadriceps is

133

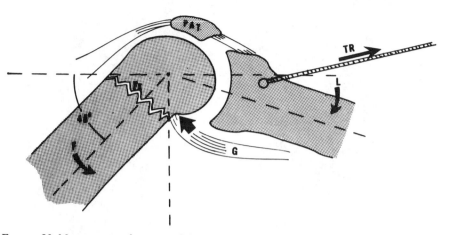

FIGURE 96. Management of supracondylar fracture. The hip is flexed 45°. The lower leg, by its weight, reduces the lower femoral fragment assisted by manual pressure *(thick arrow)* upward against the distal fragment. Traction *(TR)* is initially applied to separate the fragments. A spica cast is applied with hip and knee flexed and the pin incorporated.

early, exercises of the isometric type (quad setting) should be started immediately and immobilization in plaster should not be kept any longer than absolutely necessary.

After removal of the spica plaster, the leg may be placed in balanced suspension and more active exercises begun. Within two to four weeks, the quadriceps should be reasonably strong and the fracture adequately healed to permit weight-bearing in a walking caliper splint. Obviously, time factors are determined by age and severity of fracture as well as patient cooperation.

When closed reduction is not possible open reduction may be necessary.

Intercondylar Fractures

These fractures of the femur (Fig. 97) may be of the Y or T type; they are more severe than supracondylar fractures. Soft tissue injury may be extensive. The fracture may be exceedingly unstable with reduction and maintenance of the reduction difficult.

Management (Fig. 98) is basically that of traction to regain the length of the femur after aspiration of the joint hemorrhage, manual or clamp manipulation to approximate the condylar fragments, plaster in the reduced position, and *immediate periodic supervised quadriceps exercises.* Post-reduction care is similar to that of supracondylar fracture. Surgical (open) reduction is often necessary to gain proper reduction and to maintain the reduction. The technique will not be detailed. Several types of internal fixation are shown in Figure 99.

134

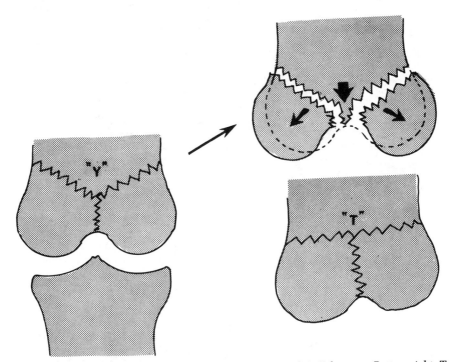

FIGURE 97. Intercondylar fractures of the distal femur. *Top left*, Y fracture. *Bottom right*, T fracture. *Top right*, Downward movement of the femur into the intercondylar fracture site separating the two condyles.

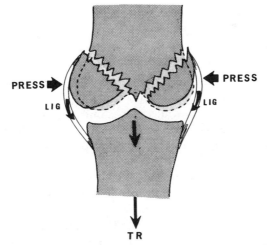

FIGURE 98. Principles of management of intercondylar femoral fracture. Traction *(TR)* elongates the femur by pulling on the collateral ligaments *(LIG)* attached to the condyles, bringing them distally where lateral and medial pressure *(PRESS)*, manually or by clamp, will approximate the fragments and reduce the fracture in order to allow casting.

135

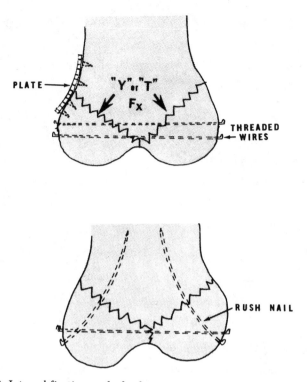

FIGURE 99. Internal fixation methods of supracondylar fractures of the distal femur.

Condylar Fractures

Condylar fractures are caused by violence, as are supracondylar and intercondylar, but usually of a different type. Whereas, supracondylar and Y or T intercondylar fractures are often caused by direct linear force, fracture of a condyle occurs from severe varus or valgus force (Fig. 100). The fracture line can be in various planes but usually is vertical and in the sagittal plane. The ligaments of the involved side usually prevent marked displacement but the ligaments of the opposite side and the cruciate ligaments are often damaged.

Management of these fractures depends exclusively on the exact repositioning of the displaced fragment(s) in order to regain continuity of the femoral surface and proper alignment with its opposing tibial surface. Closed reduction by traction and manipulation may succeed. Open reduction, using internal fixation of the fragments and repair of the involved ligaments, is often required. Status of the ligaments must be ascertained as well as careful documentation of the exact site and extent of the fractured condyle.

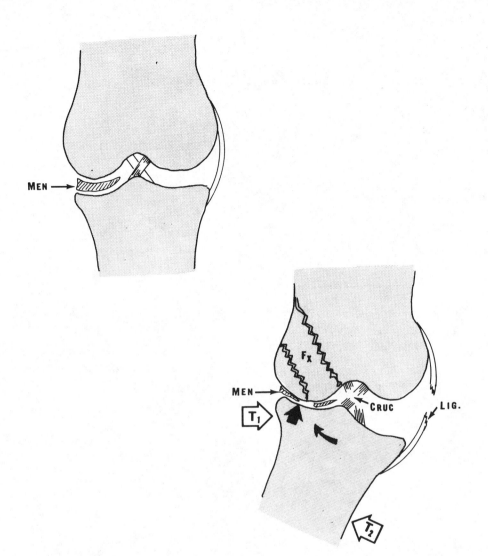

FIGURE 100. Condylar fracture from severe valgus (varus) stress. *Top,* Normal joint anatomy. *Bottom,* Force applied to the knee joint *(T₁)* or laterally to the tibia *(T₂)* can cause fracture of that condyle *(Fx)*, tear of the opposite ligament *(LIG)*, tear of either or both of the cruciate ligaments *(CRUC)*, and compression of the meniscus *(MEN)*.

Separation of the Distal Epiphysis

This occurrence may be the result of trauma and will be mentioned only briefly here. The condition occurs usually in boys between the ages of 8 and 14 years, usually from direct violence. Several types are shown in Figure 101.

137

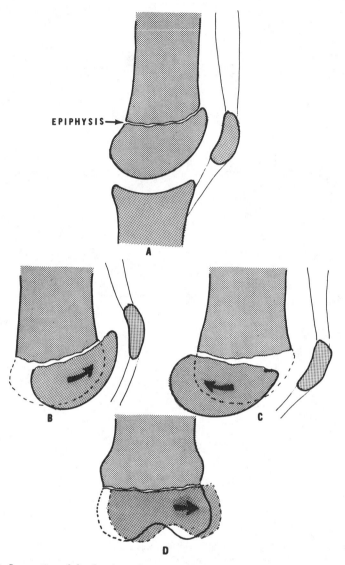

FIGURE 101. Separation of the distal epiphysis. The epiphysis can be separated dependent on the direction of the force. *A*, The normal epiphysis; *B*, The epiphysis is tilted forward; *C*, The rarer type in which the epiphysis is tilted backward; and *D*, The epiphysis may be displaced medially or laterally also.

FRACTURES OF PROXIMAL END OF TIBIA

The upper end of the tibia comprises two large condyles separated by a relatively weak bony span (Fig. 102). This fact predisposes the tibial plateau to a high incidence of fractures. The history depicts the exact mecha-

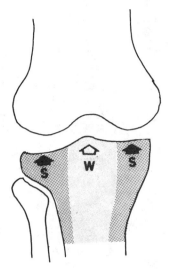

FIGURE 102. Tibial condyles: stress plates. The upper end of the tibia is comprised of two condyles: strong cortical bone (S) separated by a weaker bone span (W).

nism of the trauma causing the fracture, usually direct violence linear to the tibia or violent lateral stresses causing forceful abduction or adduction of the knee. The former is exemplified by landing on one's feet following a hard fall; the latter is exemplified by being struck from the side such as an athletic injury or being hit by a moving vehicle.

The lateral condyle is fractured more frequently than the medial and is associated with injury to the medial ligamentous structures and the cruciate ligaments. The extent of downward or lateral displacement or both is related to the force of the injury. The lateral meniscus may be crushed, forced within the comminution, or forced into the knee joint medially (Fig. 103). Severe adduction force upon the tibia (lateral force upon the knee joint) may cause fracture of the medial condyle, tear of the lateral collateral ligaments, and crushing of the medial meniscus.

Direct violence, such as a fall on extended legs, can cause vertical fracture of the tibial plateau in a Y or T fracture (Fig. 104). The ligaments may remain intact or be individually or singly injured. The center fragment may project into the fracture site and cause varying degrees of deformity. Effusion of the joint with blood is usual as these fractures are intra-articular in nature.

Management demands complete evaluation of the mechanism of fracture, relationship of the residual fragments, ligamentous injury, and the sequelae of soft tissue injuries. The aim of treatment is to restore the articular surfaces to their anatomic relationships, that is, restoration of the tibial plateau articular surface, proper relationship to the femoral condyles, restoration of ligamentous integrity, evacuation of any intra-articular debris, and restoration of quadriceps strength.

139

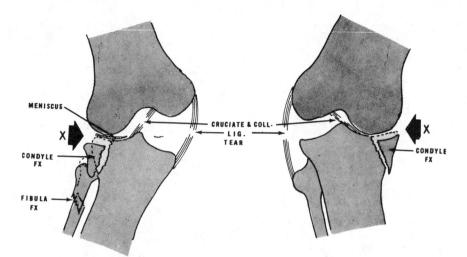

FIGURE 103. Fracture of the lateral tibial condyle. Lateral stress or uneven direct force can cause depressed fracture of the lateral condyle, crushed lateral meniscus, tear of cruciate ligaments, and tear of the medial collateral ligaments.

Management of fracture of the lateral tibial condyle begins with aspiration of hemarthrosis. If there is no displacement start active quadriceps exercises after application of a snugfitting *unpadded* plaster cast with knee in full extension. In two weeks, a new plaster is applied that remains an additional two weeks when flexion exercises are begun. Weight bearing is usually permitted in 10 to 12 weeks although crutch ambulation without weight bearing is started much sooner.

If the lateral fragment is separated and depressed after the joint is aspirated, traction along the line of the tibia is applied (Fig. 105) with

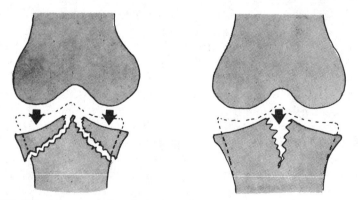

FIGURE 104. Direct trauma to the tibial plateau. Direct trauma, such as a fall on extended legs, can cause a *Y* or *T* fracture of the plateau.

140

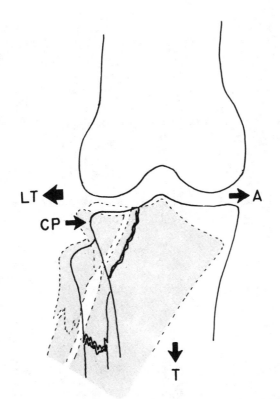

Figure 105. Principles of treatment of tibial plateau fracture. Aspirate *(A)* the hemarthrosis or effusion; apply traction *(T)*; apply lateral traction *(LT)* to cause varus and open the lateral aspect of the joint; compression *(CP)* against fragment to reduce fracture, which can be done manually or with a clamp. Cast with snug plaster.

simultaneous lateral traction applied by a large bandage passing about the medial aspect of the knee to cause varus of the knee. This last maneuver causes the lateral collateral ligament to pull up on the tibial fragment and reduce the separation. Direct pressure by the surgeon on the fragment will further reduce the depression. A compression clamp may be used by an experienced surgeon. Medial depressed tibial fractures are treated in a similar manner with the forces applied in the opposite transverse direction to cause knee *valgus*.

After reduction, the leg is casted and exercises begun as stated. The cast is kept on for eight weeks with weight bearing possible in 10 to 12 weeks, preferably *without* a knee brace if the quadriceps is sufficiently strong.

In a severely comminuted fracture, the fragments may be avascular and result in asceptic necrosis. The fragments may wedge the separated fragments and prevent close opposition. If the fragments remain separated and the surface margin irregular, degenerative arthritis, far more severe than normally expected, may result. Tears in the cartilage become filled with fibrous tissue and may create an adequate weight-bearing surface with full range of motion.

If immediate reduction is not attainable, prolonged traction in a Bohler-Braun splint using 10 to 12 lb of traction may be beneficial for reduction. If closed reduction is not possible, open reduction with internal fixation after reduction may be necessary. These indications and techniques are well documented in orthopedic literature.

FRACTURES OF THE PATELLA

Fractures of the patella have been discussed in detail in Chapter 5. Please refer to that section of text.

BIBLIOGRAPHY

OLERUD, S: *Operative treatment of supracondylar-condylar fractures of the femur.* J Bone Joint Surg 54-A:1015, 1972.

CHAPTER 8

Congenital and Acquired Deformities of the Knee

The term "congenital" implies its presence at or before birth and such deformities are common in the musculoskeletal system. They may be grouped into various categories:

1. Failure of tissue differentiation such as failure of cartilage to progress into bone.
2. Failure of fusion as exemplified in bipartite patella.
3. Supernumerary parts.
4. Deformity in the bone itself such as osteogenesis imperfecta or congenital bowing.

Bone dysplasia is considered to be a congenital variance as well as being biochemic, hormonal, and metabolic. These dystrophies and dysplasias are well documented (Stelling and Rubin). Most are rare and few affect the knee singly, but in the generalized involvement of the child the knee may also be included. *Dysplasia* (Rubin) is described as a disturbance in bone development and is *intrinsic* to bone. *Dystrophy* is defective bone development caused by *extrinsic* factors such as metabolic or nutritional abnormalities. *Dysostosis* is abnormal bone development caused by a *defect* in ectodermal or mesenchymal tissues.

In all three conditions, the extremities usually are deformed and shortened, and cause abnormal gait. The knee, besides involvement in length of the extremity, may be varus or valgus.

Genu valgum, genu varum, genu recurvatum, and tibial or femoral torsion are the most frequent deformities noted in childhood that cause parental concern over abnormal gait. Although they usually are congenital or familial they may be acquired following injury or disease or may be secondary to systemic disease.

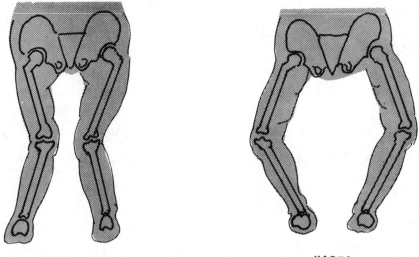

VALGUS   VARUS

FIGURE 106. Genu valgus and genu varus. *Left*, Genu valgus with the knees close to each other and the ankles separated. *Right*, Genu varus showing knees separated and ankles together.

GENU VALGUM

Genu valgum is an angular deformity of the leg, otherwise termed knock-knee, in which the ankles are separated when the knees are in contact (Fig. 106). This condition is frequently noted in childhood and there is a large familial tendency. It is often associated with severely pronated feet and in overweight children who begin ambulation at an early age. It may be secondary to rickets or fractures of the femur; caused by trauma to the epiphyseal plate, paralysis by lower motor neuron disease, cerebral palsy, or a hip defect; or idiopathic. It is frequently noted from ages two to six and is of concern when it persists to a significant degree after age six.

Prognosis depends on the etiologic factors. When the malleoli are less than three inches apart conservative treatment or natural development usually ends in good results. Conservative treatment consists of correcting the foot pronation with an inner wedge of a stiff one-eighth inch counter in shoes, weight loss, and passive stretching exercises administered by the parents.

In a severe genu valgus, surgery consists of stapling or osteotomy planned carefully depending upon the age of the child, the severity of the deformity, and the calculated growth potential (Fig. 107).

144

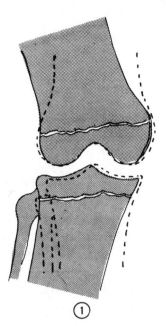

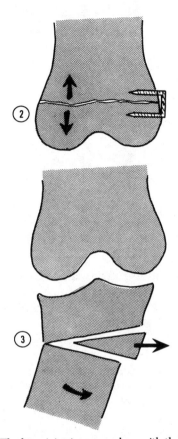

FIGURE 107. Surgical treatment of valgus or varus. *1*, The knee joint in genu valgus with the open epiphyseal line of the distal femur and proximal tibia. *2*, Stapling in which the growth on the convex side is stopped, permitting continued growth on the other side *(arrows)* with stapling held until alignment is achieved. *3*, Osteotomy of the tibia in which a wedge is removed to permit the distal portion's being brought under the proximal portion and the leg realigned.

GENU VARUM

Genu varum is an alignment abnormality of the leg in which the knees are widely separated while the ankle malleoli are in contact. This condition is commonly called bowlegs.

All normal babies at birth and during infancy have some degree c genu varum. The condition frequently persists during the first three years. Much of the varus is apparent rather than actual as a result of the normal distribution of thigh fat, the position of the legs caused by the interposition of thick diapers, and early weight bearing in chubby children. The

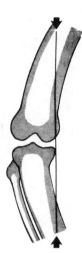

FIGURE 108. X-ray evidence of cortical thickening in valgus. It is on the concave side as a result of stress of weight bearing.

condition is aggravated by the coexistence of tibial torsion. Physiologic bowing is symmetrical and involves both femur and tibia; x-ray films show cortical thickening of the medial side of the bones (Fig. 108). Although most genu varum is physiologically caused, it may be the result of vitamin D deficiency from renal rickets or resistant dietary rickets, osteochondritits (Blount's disease), dyschondroplasia, osteogenesis imperfecta, epiphyseal injury, or neurofibromatosis.

Proper diagnosis is mandatory for proper treatment, but certain principles affect the results of any treatment. It is usually desirable to avoid precipitous early walking, insure proper bed position during sleeping, avoid excessive diapering, and institute gentle manipulative exercises by the parents. Braces are advocated for the moderate deformity that persists in later childhood (Fig. 109) or when very severe surgical intervention may be required such as stapling procedures or osteotomy. If the child is walking, a shoe correction aids in realigning the superincumbent leg. In varus, an outer wedge on the shoe of one-eighth to one-fourth inch is prescribed (Fig. 110). The efficacy of this is not confirmed.

TIBIAL TORSION

This condition may coexist with genu varus and genu valgus or be present alone. Tibial torsion in children designates torsion (twist) in the bone (tibia) in the coronal plane causing the medial malleolus to lie in a different plane than the lateral malleolus. If there is internal torsion, the medial malleolus is behind the lateral. This condition exists in the fetus but at birth the malleoli are equal. By walking age, 20° of external rotation is considered normal. More recent studies (Khermosh) indicate that

146

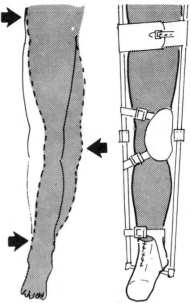

FIGURE 109. Brace treatment of valgus. A long leg brace can be constructed, which places three points of pressure *(arrows)* to correct valgus (or varus in reversed manner).

newborns have external rotation of 2.2° with gradual external torsion angle of 1.3° per year. Many investigators and clinicians deny the presence of tibial torsion in either direction. Most often tibial torsion is a self-limiting physiologic condition and may be a result of internal or external rotation of the hip. Internal tibial torsion is frequently associated with bowing, metatarsus varus, or talipes equinovarus (clubfoot). External rotation is often associated with knock-knee deformity.

If mild and not of significant cosmetic concern, no treatment is needed. Functional impairment at the worst is an abnormal gait and, in childhood, tripping over one's own feet. Treatment consists of manipulative exercises done by the parents and shoe corrections to build up the inner or outer aspect of the sole, heel, or both to cause either inversion or eversion as the condition dictates. Denis-Browne splints are advocated by some but considered useless and unphysiologic by others in so far as the stress of the splint seems to be expended to rotate the knee and not the tibial torsion (Fig. 111). Twisters may be prescribed but their value is questionable. The likelihood of their correcting torsion is limited and there is the possibility that twisters may create or aggravate knee valgus as a result of their stress (Fig. 112).

TIBIAL VARUM

Angular deformities can occur in any plane but the majority are in the coronal (valgus or varus) or in the saggital plane (recurvatum). A form of

147

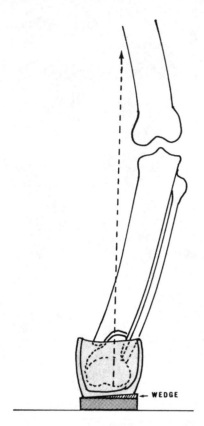

FIGURE 110. Shoe wedge treatment of genu varus. In an attempt to realign the weight-bearing stress on the knee, a sole and heel wedge may be prescribed for the outer border of the shoe. The efficacy of this is not confirmed.

← WEDGE

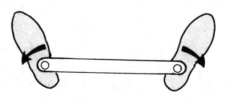

DENIS - BROWNE SPLINT

FIGURE 111. Denis-Browne night splints. The Denis-Browne splint is a pair of shoes for varus or valgus of the foot. The shoes are separated in specific degree of rotation by bending the bar. The length of the bar is equal to the desired separation of the legs as is the degree of external rotation. The bar places rotatory stress at the knee and may not be influential upon the tibial torsion.

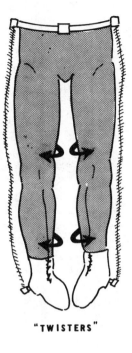

"TWISTERS"

FIGURE 112. Twister braces. Attached to a pelvic band and fixed to the shoe, the twister brace is a set of bilateral spring cables in a housing that tends to externally rotate the leg. The main value of this brace appears to be in the training of inversion gait toward more external rotation. Its static correction is doubtful.

tibia varum resulting from osteochondrosis (osteochondrosis deformans tibia or Blount's disease) requires separate discussion from the so-called physiologic bowing. In osteochondrosis deformans, there is disturbance of growth involving the metaphysis epiphysial cartilage and the osseous center of the epiphysis. The pathologic conditions are located on the medial side of the proximal tibial epiphysis causing an abrupt varus angular deformity (Fig. 113). The condition may be unilateral but 50 percent of the cases are bilateral.

The criteria of osteochondrosis tibia varum are:

1. A sharp angular deformity immediately below the proximal tibial epiphysis.
2. An irregular epiphysial cartilage.
3. A wedge-shaped osseous portion of the epiphysis.
4. A beak projection forming from the medial metaphysis.
5. Lax medial ligaments.

Onset usually is insidious. If bilateral, the child develops a waddle gait; if the condition is unilateral the child develops a limp. Clinically, the leg reveals a sharp angular deformity below the knee. Treatment is expectant

149

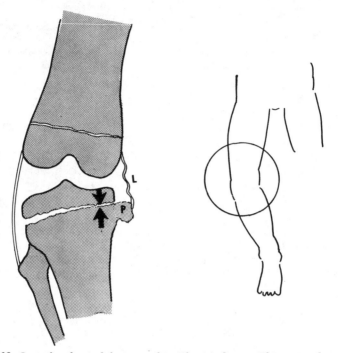

FIGURE 113. Osteochondrosis deformans tibia: Blount's disease. This entity, described by W. Blount, is medial osteochondrosis with sharp angular deformity immediately below the proximal tibial epiphysis, an irregular medial cartilage, the medial metaphysis forming a beak-like projection *(P)* and lax medial ligaments *(L)*.

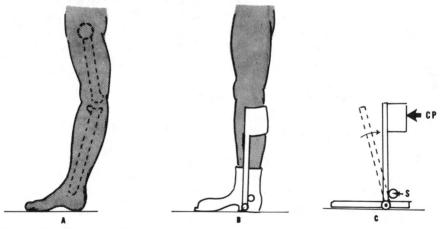

FIGURE 114. Treatment of genu recurvatum by short leg brace. A brace with a down-stop at the ankle. By decreasing equinus and thus secondary back knee, it may be effective in preventing recruvatum. *C*, Mechanical principle of the brace: the stop *(S)*; calf pressure *(CP)*; and the allowable excursion *(curved arrow)* of the upright bars of the brace on the fixed foot to the floor.

150

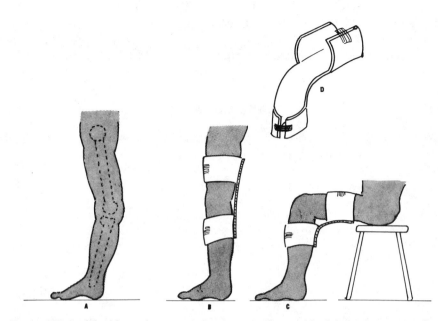

FIGURE 115. Back heel brace for genu recurvatum. *A*, The usual back knee stance, regardless of numerous etiologic factos. Brace designed to control recurvatum in standing *(B)* and to permit sitting *(C)*. *D*, The brace is a dynamic splint made of orthoplast with 25° flexion molded into splint. (Adapted from Andersen, CB: *Dynamic knee splint to prevent hyperextension.* Phys Ther 52:944, 1972.)

and conservative because spontaneous correction does occur. Since this deformity does not progress after the epiphysis (cartilage) is closed, operative intervention for correction probably should be deferred until closure is ascertained.

GENU RECURVATUM

Genu recurvatum has numerous causes ranging from intrinsic pathologic conditions of the knee to secondary factors. The most common cause is fixed plantar flexion from either contracture (of numerous etiologies) or spastic equinus. Excessive compensation of the quadriceps plus weak gastrocnemius soleus may be causative. (See Chapter 9 on gait for explanation.) Excessive gluteal contractions with no soleus or quadriceps may also cause recurvatum.

Treatment is based on correction of the etiologic factor(s) and may consist of exercises to regain muscle balance or to stretch the offending contracture. Serial casts may be applied. It is important to consider surgical release of the offending muscle-tendons *before* excessive changes occur. A brace with an ankle down-stop may be useful (Fig. 114); this may

151

be incorporated with a back knee stop that simultaneously permits knee flexion for walking and sitting. The knee portion of the brace that prevents back knee also applies pressure to aid proprioception at the pressure sites (Fig. 115).

BIBLIOGRAPHY

ANDERSEN, CB: *Dynamic knee splint to prevent hyperextension*. Phys Ther 52:944, 1972.

BLOUNT, WP: *Tibia vara*. J Bone Joint Surg 19:1, 1937.

HUTTER, CG AND SCOTT, W: *Tibial torsion*. J Bone Joint Surg 31-A:511, 1949.

KHERMOSH, O, LIOR, G, AND WEISSMAN, SL: *Tibial torsion in children*. Clin Orthop 79:25, 1971.

KLEVEN, DK, PERRY, J, AND HISLOP, H: *The ankle joint: An anatomical and mechanical study using amputated specimens*. Thesis, Los Angeles, 1970.

MAJESTRO, TC AND FROST, HM: *Posterior transposition of the origins of the anatomic internal rotators of the hip*. Clin Orthop 79:57, 1971.

PERRY, J: *Bracing the knee*. J Canad Physiotherap Assoc 24:198, 1972.

RUBIN, P: *Dynamic Classification of Bone Dysplasia*. Year Book Medical Publishers, Chicago, 1964.

SMITH, EM AND JUVINALL, RR: *Mechanics of bracing*. In LICHT, S (ED): *Orthotics Etcetera*. Licht, New Haven, 1966.

STELLING, FH: *General affection of the skeletal system*. Pediatr Clin North Am 14:359, 1967.

CHAPTER 9

The Knee in Gait: Normal and Abnormal

The functional knee in stance and in gait in childhood and adulthood must be understood before specifics of the abnormal gait and stance can be evaluated and remedied. Factors to be considered are (1) quadriceps competency, (2) neuromuscular incoordination, (3) limitation of range of motion, (4) proprioception adequacy, and (5) relationship and adequacy of contiguous joints (hip, ankle, or both). All must be taken into consideration in evaluating proper knee function or its relative dysfunction.

NORMAL GAIT

In the normal gait, the trunk shifts from side to side with approximately 2 cm of displacement. This motion attempts to minimize vertical body displacement to decrease energy expenditure. This trunk shift, laterally and rotatory, requires precise external muscular control and delicate proprioception. The total body weight above the pelvis consists of: trunk, 50 percent of total body weight; head, 8 percent; each upper extremity, 8 percent; and during the swing phase the swinging leg, 15 percent. At the one-leg stance during gait, 85 percent of the total body weight must be balanced.

The *swing phase* is initially to advance the limb preparatory to heel strike of the stance phase. The hip flexes 20° and the knee 60°. At mid-swing, the knee remains slightly flexed with the ankle dorsiflexed to clear the floor. At the end of the swing phase the knee becomes fully extended (Fig. 116). The *stance phase* begins immediately upon the swinging leg striking the floor ahead of the body. The heel contacts the floor and the knee flexes slightly to dampen the impact—approximately 15°. At mid-stance, as the foot becomes flat upon the floor, the knee gradually extends and remains extended throughout the remainder of the stance phase until at the pre-swing the knee flexes to 35° (Fig. 117).

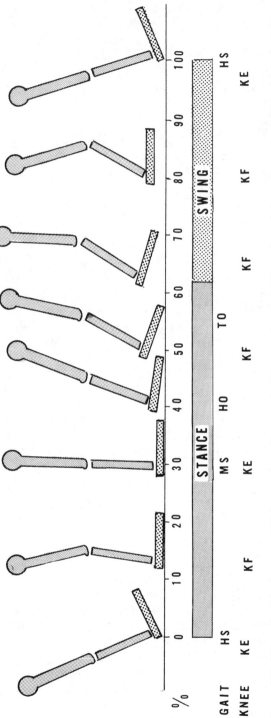

FIGURE 116. Gait cycle. The percentage (%) denotes the increments of a full gait cycle—in this figure the right leg in one cycle. *HS* is heel strike beginning the stance phase (62%). At heel strike, the knee is extended (*KE*). As the body passes over the weight-bearing leg, the knee flexes slightly (*KF*) to absorb shock. At mid-stance (*MS* 30%), the knee is extended (*KE*). At heel-off (*HO* 40%), the knee begins to flex slightly (*KF* 50%) and remains flexed through toe-off (*TO* 62%) when the swing phase begins. The knee remains flexed throughout swing phase until pre-heel strike when the knee re-extends (*KE* 100%).

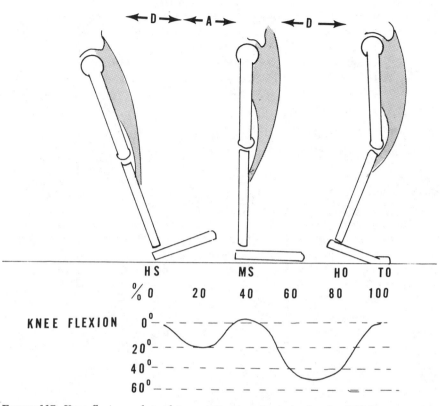

FIGURE 117. Knee flexion and quadriceps action in gait. At heel strike *(HS)* beginning the stance phase *(0%)*, the quadricpes is contracted then decelerates *(D)* as it flexes. At mid-stance *(MS 40%)*, the quadriceps has actively extended the knee *(A)*. As the stance phase progresses, the knee again flexes, but more (to 60°), and again the quadriceps decelerates flexion. After toe-off *(TO 100%)*, the leg is in swing phase and quadriceps actively extends the knee and swings the leg forward. The stickman figures here are not directly above the graphs or the numerals.

The muscular action upon the knee is as follows. At the initiation of the swing, the short head of the biceps (hamstrings), the gracilis, and the sartorius contract. During the mid-swing, the knee acts mechanically without muscular action until the end of the swing phase when the quadriceps contracts to extend the knee preparatory to heel strike. The quadriceps may act at the hip joint to flex the hip and begin the swing. At heel strike (the beginning of the stance phase), the quadriceps contracts to maintain knee extension and prepare for mid-stance phase when the knee flexes to absorb the impact and decrease the vertical arc of the pelvis in forward translation.

During the swing phase, the pelvis internally rotates. The femur internally rotates upon the pelvis and the tibia internally rotates upon the femur. This internal rotation continues through the first 20 percent of the stance phase but as mid-stance phase is approached the pelvis begins to externally rotate and the femur externally rotates upon the pelvis and the tibia upon the femur until the beginning of the swing phase (Fig. 118).

This rotation of the entire leg is also accompanied by pronation and supination of the foot. At heel strike the foot is supinated; becomes pronated at mid-stance, continues to pronate during stance to again supinate at toe off, the beginning of the swing phase (Fig. 119). During the time that the foot is flat (approximately 7 to 45 percent of stance phase), the thigh is rotating externally—about 10°. As the foot, during this phase is plantigrade (flat) and not rotating, the thigh rotation is absorbed at the knee. The femur rotates approximately 6°, the tibia 9 to 10°, thus, there also is some rotational torque at the knee.

The hamstrings become active at the end of the swing phase (Fig. 120). As they elongate during the swing phase, they decelerate the swinging leg. They probably also initiate or assist in flexing the knee as the leg goes into heel strike (HS). At heel off (HO) at the end of the stance phase, they passively flex (deceleration) the leg that is now going through the swing phase.

At heel strike, the hip extensors bring the body forward above the weight-bearing leg (Fig. 121). The knee of the striking leg maintains a slight knee flexion (10 to 15°) to dampen the impact. If there is hip extensor weakness, the pelvis moves ahead (further) over the center of gravity and further flexes the knee (see Fig. 121), which causes the femur to be more horizontal and thus creates more stress upon the weight-bearing quadriceps. Good hip extensors and good proprioceptive sense will extend the hip and pull the thigh over the fixed lower leg and foot and thus impose less stress upon the quadriceps. During this gait phase (heel strike to stance phase) over the fixed foot, the lower leg must achieve stability with adequate ankle plantar flexors.

A weak soleus, or a gait in which the soleus for push-off is not effective, permits the knee to flex during the stance gait (Fig. 122). In a foot that has a contracted soleus group (contracture or neurologic spasticity), the plantar flexed (fixed) foot mechanically extends the knee as the pelvis passes over the center of gravity (Fig. 123). Contracture of the posterior knee tissues, causing a flexed knee, places excessive stress upon the quadriceps and can be assisted by strong hip extensor and ankle plantar flexor groups. Fifteen degrees of flexion can be accepted if the ankle and hip musculature is strong enough to compensate for the flexure (Fig. 124). A hip flexion contracture also flexes the weight-bearing knee and can be balanced by adequate quadriceps and soleus. The forward flexed posture, where the upper body brings the center of gravity ahead of the knee (see Fig. 124), places stress on all the leg extensors.

156

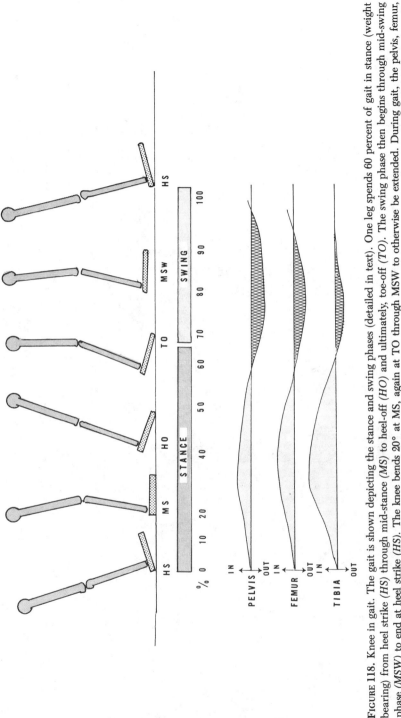

FIGURE 118. Knee in gait. The gait is shown depicting the stance and swing phases (detailed in text). One leg spends 60 percent of gait in stance (weight bearing) from heel strike (HS) through mid-stance (MS) to heel-off (HO) and ultimately, toe-off (TO). The swing phase then begins through mid-swing phase (MSW) to end at heel strike (HS). The knee bends 20° at TO through MSW to otherwise be extended. During gait, the pelvis, femur, and tibia, each slightly independent, undergo internal rotation (IN) during stance phase as the body passes over the weight-bearing leg. Just before the beginning of the swing phase (50%) and through the swing phase, the pelvis, femur, and tibia externally rotate (OUT) the tibia more than the femur. Rotatory torque occurs at the knee.

157

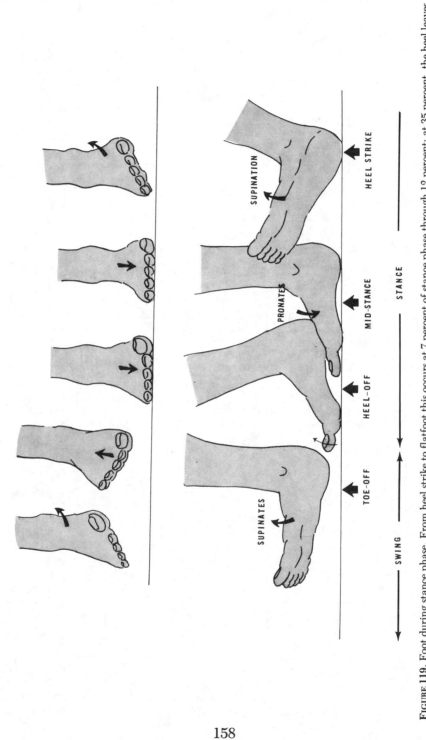

FIGURE 119. Foot during stance phase. From heel strike to flatfoot this occurs at 7 percent of stance phase through 12 percent; at 35 percent, the heel leaves the floor (heel-off). Toe-off starts the swing phase of that leg and begins at 60 percent of stance phase.

158

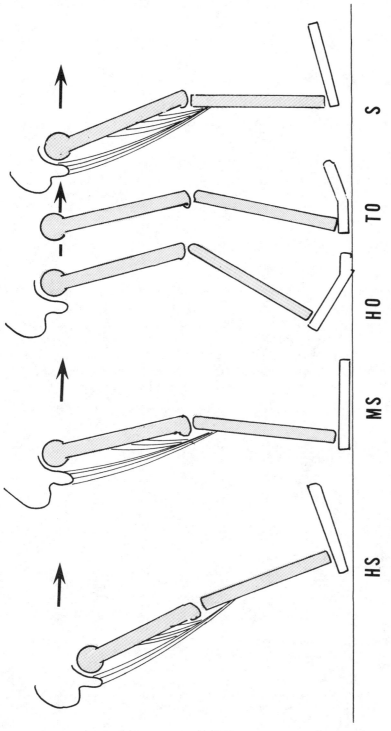

FIGURE 120. Action of hamstrings in gait. The hamstrings decelerate the leg at the termination of the swing phase (S) prior to heel strike (HS). During stance phase at mid-point (MS), the hamstrings presumably assist in hip extension.

159

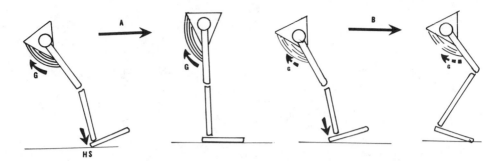

FIGURE 121. Gait analysis. *A*, Normal gait with heel strike *(HS)*, the knee slightly flexed to dampen the impact. The hip extensors *(G)* extend the hip and pull the pelvis over the weight-bearing leg at the stance phase. *B*, Gait with weak gluteal (hip) extensors *(G)* that fail to extend the hip, and thus at stance phase the knee is still flexed as the pelvis passes over the fixed foot. *Right*, The foot is in equinus stance and is not related to the hip weakness.

Patients with weak knee extensors (quadriceps) *and* weak hip extensors can lean the trunk backward in order to balance over their center of gravity. This requires good proprioception and muscle control.

Weak ankle plantar flexors can cause knee instability since the quadriceps does not contract quickly enough to prevent tripping or knee buckling. Loss of proprioception also can contribute to the condition. A short leg brace that controls plantar flexion *or* dorsiflexion may be needed to improve gait. The type of brace is determined by careful gait analysis.

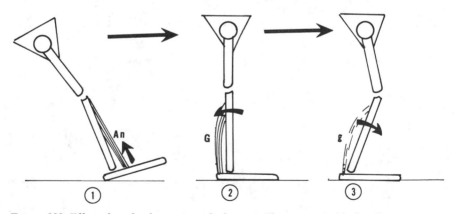

FIGURE 122. Effect of weak soleus gait on the knee. *1*, The anticus (ankle dorsiflexor) *(An)* at heel strike prevents foot slap. *2*, As the pelvis passes over the fixed foot during stance phase the gastrocnemius-soleus muscle *(G)* prevents excessive ankle dorsiflexion and decelerates the leg as it passes over the fixed foot. This action simultaneously prevents the knee from flexing in stance. *3*, With a weak soleus *(g)* excessive ankle dorsiflexion occurs and the knee flexes unless strong quadriceps or strong hip extensors or both intervene.

160

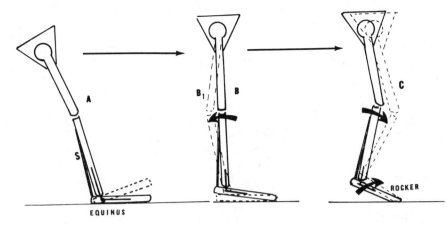

EQUINUS

FIGURE 123. Equinus gait: contracted or spastic soleus. A, There is no heel strike because the foot in in equinus during the swing phase. B, Normally extended knee. As the pelvis passes over the fixed foot the shortened soleus extends the knee mechanically. If the equinus is excessive, *(B₁)*, back knee (hyperextension) can occur *(broken line)*. C, In a marked equinus during the last part of the stance phase, the foot can rock over the weight-bearing toes and throw the pelvis ahead of the center of gravity. This imposes marked stress upon the quadriceps or permits falling if the quadriceps is inadequate.

Patients suffering from flaccid paralysis (for example, peripheral neuropathy, amyotrophic lateral sclerosis, polio), who have good proprioception can accommodate well to their paresis. With impaired proprioception such as in myelomeningoceles or with poor motor control as in cerebral palsy and stroke, compensatory gait is difficult to achieve. Children with myelomeningocele usually lack strong gastrocnemius-soleus muscles as well as hip extensors *and* have impaired sensory level. Loss of proprioception or loss of motor control may be an indication for bracing.

CONCLUSION

Careful evaluation of the function or malfunction of the knee requires:

1. Neurologic examination for motor, spastic, or flaccid paresis and proprioception.
2. Orthopedic evaluation for contracture or malalignment.
3. Careful stance and gait evaluation.

Upon performance of all these tests and careful evaluation of their significance, proper treatment can be prescribed; be it exercise, bracing, or surgery. Failure of definitive treatment can be related to improper evaluation more often than to faulty treatment technique.

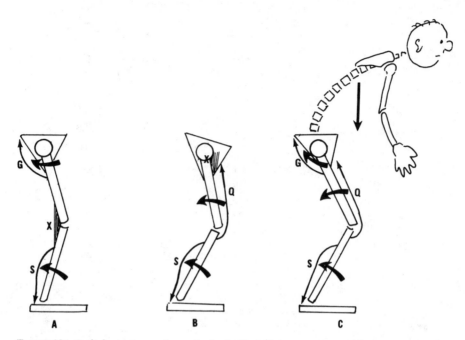

FIGURE 124. Pathologic stance phase of gait. *A,* Flexed knee stance caused by contracture *(X)* of the knee. Erect stance is possible with strong hip extensors *(G,* gluteals) and strong plantar flexors *(S,* soleus). *B,* Flexed stance as a result of hip flexion contracture *(X)* overcome by strong quadriceps *(Q)* and strong soleus *(S).* The former extends the knee and the latter pulls the leg back over the fixed foot. *C,* Flexed stance resulting from bent-over posture with most of the body weight (60 to 65 percent) placed ahead of the center of gravity. All extensors are needed to maintain erect stance.

BIBLIOGRAPHY

BASMAJIAN, JV: *Muscles Alive. Their Function Revealed by Electromyography.* Williams & Wilkins, Baltimore, 1962.

INMAN, VT, RALSTON, HJ, AND TODD, F: *Human Walking.* Williams & Wilkins, Baltimore, 1981.

LEVENS, AS, INMAN, VT, AND BLOSSER, JA: *Transverse rotation of the segments of the lower extremity in locomotion.* J Bone Joint Surg 30-A:859, 1948.

LIBERSON, WT: *Biomechanics of gait: A method of study.* Archives of Physical Medicine 46:37, 1965.

MURRAY, MP, DROUGHT, AB, AND KORY, RC: *Walking patterns of normal men.* J Bone Joint Surg 46-A:335, 1964.

PERRY, J: *Bracing of the knee.* Journal of the Canadian Physical Therapy Association 24:298, 1972.

SAUNDERS, JB DE CM, INMAN, VT, AND EBERHART, HD: *Major determinants in normal and pathological gait.* J Bone Joint Surg 35-A:543, 1953.

SCHENKER, AW: *Pathological implications of abnormal stance and gait. Occupational Therapy and Rehabilitation* 28:131, 1949.

CHAPTER 10

The Knee in Cerebral Palsy

The knee is involved in most types of cerebral palsy as a result of muscle imbalance or secondary to hip or foot-ankle deviation, contracture, or surgical intervention. The goals of treatment of cerebral palsy are to develop and utilize to potential that which is not present as a result of central nervous system damage before, at, or after birth. Treatment is thus to correct defect when possible, prevent new defects that may occur, improve the remaining capacities, and prevent unwanted substitutions but simultaneously provide and encourage desirable substitution functions.

The child with a birth defect of the central nervous system may be born with a specific type of defect but this defect or its disability may change during the subsequent stages of development from early weeks of life. The exact type of defect and its resultant disability often varies with each examination.

Ambulation receives priority in considering the evaluation and stress of treatment. Hand dexterity and communication *should* receive priority but ambulation is demanded by the parents. Numerous forms of treatment have had their claimants in the treatment of cerebral palsy: intracranial cortical surgical ablation, cranial blood vessel ligation, cord tracheotomies, ventral root or dorsal root surgery, and alcohol or phenol nerve blocks to alter the neuromuscular abnormality, imbalance, or incoordination. No surgical procedure, be it upon the central nervous system, peripheral nervous system, or any aspect of the musculoskeletal system, alters the underlying abnormal pattern(s) of movement. The main benefit of surgical procedure is prevention or alteration of deformity and improvement of function, appearance, or both.

Treatment by exercise aims to improve strength, balance, and coordination and increase range of articular motion. In cerebral palsy, classification of the hypotonic or athetoid child is not of concern regarding joint limitation, but this is a concern in the spastic or tension patient. In this latter category, the concern is more of contracture of the legs in the hip

163

flexors (adductors), hamstrings, and the gastrocnemius-soleus muscle groups. Exercises to stretch these groups, when instituted early, persistently, and correctly, may be effective. If all these criteria are met and, with combined proper use of splinting, the limitation persists or progresses, surgical intervention, such as muscle-tendon transplantation or release, or both, should be given serious consideration.

Exercises obviously are limited in their application as to duration, intensity, frequency, and tolerance by the patient and the therapist or parents. Properly prescribed and fitted night splints or braces will have definite value to maintain the gains made by judicious daytime exercises. At the present time, drugs given parenterally or orally have proven disappointing.

Evaluation of the cerebral palsied patient may mislead the unwary or unskilled examiner in the interpretation of weakness of specific muscle groups with inadequate function when the weakness is essentially comparative weakness of agonist pitted against an unyielding overwhelming spastic antagonist. Release of this opposing antagonist may often re-strengthen the alleged weak ineffectual agonist and functional improvement may result.

The child with cerebral palsy must first develop head and neck balance before any further antigravity function can be expected. This must be followed by improved trunk control used in sitting balance. Hand and arm function are required before the next stage, standing balance, can be sought and achieved. Gait evolves after standing balance by acquiring strength, agonist-antagonist balance, and reciprocal movement.

Numerous techniques of physiotherapy are available to train the child in better neck and head balance, sitting trunk balance, and standing balance. Standing balance is aided by support within a mechanical apparatus that encircles the patient. This is followed by support from a wall behind the child; from which the child gradually progresses to unassisted balance. At first, stance is begun with wide based footing while standing between parallel bars. The child progresses to canes with a wide base (weighted or not, as indicated) and then gait training. The use of a walker delays development of balance. Excessive bracing that denies all undesired motions is also questioned and probably better avoided. Each stage of function and each stage of development must be re-evaluated. The treatment of the neuromuscularly defective child is not static and each stage must be ascertained.

Since the subject of this book is the knee, this specific joint must be evaluated although the remainder of the child must not be ignored. Knee function depends upon stress factors imparted upon it by the foot-ankle position, balance of the tonus of the opposing flexors and extensors, contracture of the periarticular soft tissues, and coordinated neuromuscular action of all the muscles about the knee, the foot-ankle, the hip, and the superincumbent trunk.

164

In athetosis, which constitutes 25 percent of cerebral palsy cases, braces may be used in the lower extremity essentially for *training,* not for correction or prevention of contracture. Braces are of no value in the ataxic form of cerebral palsy; in this condition skis, weighted shoes, square heels on the shoes, and physiotherapy exercises are of value. Braces applied to the lower extremity may be used to direct specific motion and prevent unwanted motion but their value in this approach is questioned by many physicians.

A deforming condition, which occurs in the spastic type of cerebral palsy, is spastic internal femoral torsion. This consists of internal rotation of the distal femur in relation to the proximal femur. Clinically, although the patella points straight ahead when the patient is standing or lying supine, the patella points (rotates) inward when the patient walks. This is frequently concomitant with associated internal tibial torsion, compensatory external tibial torsion, or genu valgum that allow the feet to point directly ahead during gait. Internal femoral torsion owing to spasticity appears when the child begins walking between ages 1.5 to 2.0 years and becomes stable at maturity with no further progression.

Related etiologically to spastic internal femoral torsion is adductor spasticity with the child becoming erect in a spastic crouch posture. The adductors are not *normally* internal rotators but when the knees are held in the flexed position as in the crouch posture and the foot *fixed* to the floor (weight bearing), the adductors become internal rotators (Fig. 125).

In the crouch posture during gait at heel strike, there is an adductor twist, which simulates internal rotation. If this condition is bilateral, a scissoring gait results. In this gait owing to spasticity at heel strike, the tensor fascia femoris and the gluteus minimus *overcontract* and add to internal rotation of the hip.

The commonly used twister brace (see Fig. 112), to eliminate internal rotation during gait, may aggravate the rotation and intensify the valgus knee posture with minimal temporary benefit and *no* permanent recovery. Treatment is best initiated by adductor tenotomy and neurectomy of the anterior branch of the obturator nerve done *extrapelvicly.* If the internal rotation and scissoring are severe, consideration must be given to stripping the origin of the tensor fascia femoris and the gluteus minimus, which now, in the crouch posture, are functionally internal rotators. The procedure is to roll posteriorly the anterior origin from the iliac crest and bifurcate it to the capsule of the hip capsule. By this posterior move, the line of pull is that of *external* rotation, at least removing its *internal* rotatory pull.

There are several basic indications of surgery (Eggers):

1. Elimination or diminution of an unwanted muscle function by procedures such as neurectomy.
2. Alteration of function of a muscle group such as causing a flexor to become an extensor.

165

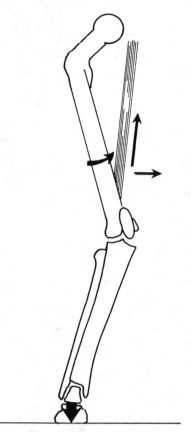

FIGURE 125. Internal femoral torsion from adductor mechanism. When the foot is fixed to the floor *(arrow)* and the knee and hip flexed in the crouch position of cerebral palsy, the adductors that act upon the leg cause valgus at the knee and internally rotate the femur. If this occurs bilaterally, the classic scissor gait results.

3. Negation by moving *part* of a muscle to cause a *biarthrodal* muscle to become a *monoarthrodal* muscle (for instance the recession of the gastrocnemius that acts across the posterior knee joint and inserting it below, thus causing its action merely at the ankle joint).

4. A negative-positive alteration, which is similar to negation, in order to transfer the hamstrings from the tibia to attach to the femur and thus decrease knee flexion (negative), improve hip extension (positive), and incidentally improve hip adduction and decrease lumbar lordosis (Fig. 126).

There are modifications to Eggers' classic procedure, dependent upon the desired result, the extent of desired correction of deforming muscle forces, and the anticipated resultant function for that particular patient.

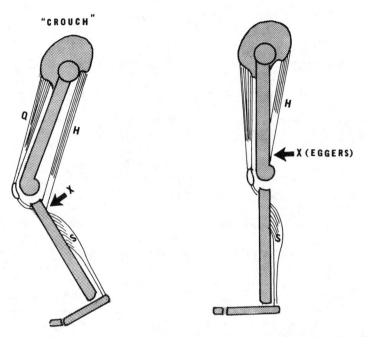

FIGURE 126. Crouch position in spastic cerebral palsy: Eggers' procedure. *Left,* Crouch posture caused by spastic hamstrings *(H)* flexing the knee. There is a simultaneous hip flexion and foot equinus. *Right,* By transplanting the hamstring insertions from the tibia to the posterior femur, knee flexion is eliminated. The hips thus extend more and the equinus is improved or corrected.

If ambulation is not anticipated, all hamstring muscles are divided to minimize flexion contracture and the resultant nursing and child care needs. If the child walks with a crouch gait but has full knee extension when recumbent, the Egger's procedure merely divides the gracilis, lengthens the semimembranosus, and transfers the semitendinosus and the biceps. If ankle equinus persists after hamstring transfer, a neurectomy of the soleus or a tendoachilles lengthening may need to be considered. The need, the extent, and the type of procedure indicated are decided with careful evaluation.

Treatment of cerebral palsy by nonsurgical measures is varied with numerous techniques, principals, methods, and equivocal results. Exercises are varied, including those intended to maintain full range of motion by passive stretching, balance the agonist with the spastic antagonists, re-educate the central nervous system by proprioceptive techniques, inhibit reflexes, utilize pathologic reflexes, and stimulate cutaneous and musculocutaneous reflexes. The basis of some of these techniques can be gleaned from the bibliography.

167

BIBLIOGRAPHY

BOBATH, K AND BOBATH, BA: *A treatment of cerebral palsy.* Brit J Phys Med 15:105, 1952.

CAILLIET, R: *Bracing for Spasticity.* In LICHT, S (ED): *Orthotics Etcetera.* Licht, New Haven, 1966.

DEAVER, GG: *Methods of treating the neuromuscular disabilities.* Archives of Physical Medicine 37:363, 1956.

EGGERS, GWN: *Transplantation of hamstring tendons to femoral condyles in order to improve hip extension and to decrease knee flexion in cerebral spastic paralysis.* J Bone Joint Surg 34-A:827, 1952.

EGGERS, GWN: *Surgical division of the patella retinacula to improve extension of the knee joint in cerebral spastic paralysis.* J Bone Joint Surg 32-A:80, 1950.

EGGERS, GWN AND EVANS, EB: *Surgery in cerebral palsy, AAOS instructional course lecture.* J Bone Joint Surg 45-A:1275, 1963.

FAY, T: *The use of pathological and unlocking reflexes in the rehabilitation of spastics.* Am J Phys Med 33:347, 1954.

GILLETTE, HE: *Kinesiology of cerebral palsy.* Clin Orthop 47:31, 1966.

KABAT, H: *Studies on neuromuscular dysfunction. XI. New principles of neuromuscular reeducation.* Permante Foundation Medical Bulletin 5:3, 1947.

KNOTT, M AND VOSS, DE: *Proprioceptive Neuromuscular Facilitation,* ed 2. Harper & Row, New York, 1968.

MAJESTRO, TC AND FROST, HM: *Cerebral palsy: Spastic internal femoral torsion.* Clin Orthop 79:44, 1971

Index

A t represents a table.
An italic number represents a figure.

169

172

meniscus
  Apley test in, 48, *50*
  arthrography in, 51-52, *53, 54*
  buckling in, 47
  clicking in, 47
  clinical meniscus signs in, 47, 48-51, *50-52*
  clinical-pathologic concepts of, 44-46, *45*
  diagnostic signs and symptoms of, 45, 46-47, *48, 49,* 51-52, *53, 54*
  effusion in, 46
  etiology of, 41-44, *43, 44*
  hyperflexion meniscus test in, 51, *52*
  incidence of, 41
  locking in, *45,* 46
  McMurray sign in, 47, *50*
  pain in, 46
  patient history in, 46
  quadriceps atrophy in, 47, *48, 49*
  Steinmann's tenderness displacement sign, 48-51, *51*
  tenderness in, 46
  tests for, 47-51, *48-52*
  treatment for
    conservative, 52-54, *55-56*
    quadriceps exercise, 57-62, *59-61*
    reduction, 52-55, *55*
    surgical, 52-54, *56-57*
  nerve, severe sprain and, 75, *77*
  rotatory knee, 66, *69*
  sprain
    severe, nerve injury and, 75, *77*
  superior tibiofibular
    extension in, 76-78, *78, 79*
    flexion in, 76-78, *78, 79*
    mechanisms of, 78
    treatment for, 80
Intercondylar fracture, 134, *135*
Internal femoral torsion
  cerebral palsy and, 165, *166*
Internal tibial torsion
  cerebral palsy and, 165

Joint(s). *See also* Ligament(s); *specific joint.*
  blood supply of, 6, *6*
  capsule, 3, *4*
  fractures about the, 131-142. *See also* Fracture(s).
  patellofemoral
    injuries and diseases, 84-106. *See also* Injury(ies).

quadriceps femoris muscle and, 84, *85*
superior tibiofibular
  function of, 76-78, *78, 79*
  injury, 78-80
surfaces
  anatomy of, structural, 1-3, *2, 3*

Knee
  anatomy of
    functional, 31-40
    structural, 1-29
  arthrides affecting the, 108-129
  cerebral palsy and, 163-167
  deformities of, 143-152
  diseases, patellar, 84-106
  gait and, 153-162
  injuries
    ligamentous-capsular, 63-82
    meniscus, 41-62
    patellar, 84-106
  joint
    blood supply of, 6, *6*
    capsule, 3, *4*
    fractures about the, 131-142
  surfaces
    anatomy of, structural, 1-3, *2, 3*
Knee-jerk reflex, 19
Knock-knee. *See* Genu valgum.

Lateral condyle fracture, 139
Lateral tibial condyle fracture, 140-142, *141*
Ligament(s). *See also* Joint(s); *specific ligament.*
  anatomy of, functional
    extension and, 39
  anterior cruciate
    anatomy of, functional, 31, *35*
  capsular
    anatomy of, functional, 34-35, *37*
  capsular and collateral
    anatomy of, functional, 31, *34*
  lateral portion of
    anatomy of, structural, 8, *10,* 12-16, *14*
  medial portion of
    anatomy of, structural, 8-12, *10-13*
  collateral
    anatomy of, functional, 36, *39*
  cruciate
    anatomy of
      functional, 36, *39*
      structural, 7, 8, *9*

173

175